# A Brief Social History of Tuberculosis

*A Brief Social History of Tuberculosis* delves into the history of tuberculosis and its impact on human populations.

Drawing on research and expert experiences, the three research chapters (Chapters 3–5) will explore how the disease has affected communities throughout history, and how society has responded to the threat of tuberculosis over time. Tuberculosis has been a persistent and devastating force from the crowded cities of the Industrial Revolution to the present day. However, this book will argue that there is much to be learned from the successes and failures of past efforts to control the disease from a social perspective. By examining the history of tuberculosis, researchers and policymakers can gain valuable insights into the challenges of infectious disease control, as well as the social and political factors that shape our response to such challenges.

This volume will focus on generating critical discussions among scholars, researchers, and policymakers; it will be informative, engaging, and an essential read for anyone interested in the history of medicine, public health, and the ongoing struggle against infectious diseases worldwide.

**Arnab Chakraborty**, College of Liberal Arts, Shanghai University, China. Arnab is a research fellow and a historian of global health, medicine, and diseases. He has conducted his research in India, the UK, the USA, the Philippines, and Fiji. Arnab's current research lies at the intersection of health policies, migration studies, and the history of medicine in non-Western societies within the context of development.

**Janaka Jayawickrama**, College of Liberal Arts, Shanghai University, China. Janaka is professor of social anthropology and has been collaborating with conflict and disaster-affected communities in Asia, Africa, and the Middle East to facilitate well-being. He has conducted frontline humanitarian responses, research, evaluations, and policy analysis for the UN, governments, and humanitarian agencies since 1994. Janaka is also the Director of the Research Centre for Health and Wellbeing.

**Yong-an Zhang,** College of Liberal Arts, Shanghai University, China. Yong-an is a professor of history and Director of the International Center for Drug Policy Studies. He has been conducting policy research from a historical perspective and focuses on their delivery for the benefit of the people.

# A Brief Social History of Tuberculosis

Key Challenges to Global Health

**Edited by
Arnab Chakraborty,
Janaka Jayawickrama, and
Yong-an Zhang**

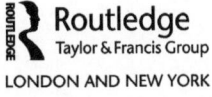

Routledge
Taylor & Francis Group

LONDON AND NEW YORK

Designed cover image: Routledge

First published 2025
by Routledge
4 Park Square, Milton Park, Abingdon, Oxon OX14 4RN

and by Routledge
605 Third Avenue, New York, NY 10158

*Routledge is an imprint of the Taylor & Francis Group, an informa business*

© 2025 selection and editorial matter, Arnab Chakraborty, Janaka Jayawickrama, and Yong-an Zhang individual chapters, the contributors

The right of Arnab Chakraborty, Janaka Jayawickrama, and Yong-an Zhang to be identified as the authors of the editorial material, and of the authors for their individual chapters, has been asserted in accordance with sections 77 and 78 of the Copyright, Designs and Patents Act 1988.

*British Library Cataloguing-in-Publication Data*
A catalogue record for this book is available from the British Library

ISBN: 978-1-032-63461-6 (hbk)
ISBN: 978-1-032-63462-3 (pbk)
ISBN: 978-1-032-63464-7 (ebk)

DOI: 10.4324/9781032634647

Typeset in Times New Roman
by codeMantra

# Contents

# Figures

# Tables

# Contributor Biographies

**Niels Brimnes** is a historian specializing in the history of colonialism and the history of global health, most often based on cases related to India and South Asia. His first monograph *Constructing the Colonial Encounter. Right and Left Hand Castes in Early Colonial South India* investigates encounters between local elites and colonial authorities in eighteenth-century South India. He also has a broad interest in the history of Danish colonialism.

**Paul H. Mason** is an Australian anthropologist with a diverse research portfolio spanning multiple continents. Mason's research extends to the social, economic, and political dimensions of tuberculosis, with publications on ethics, gender, mental health, and social models of tuberculosis. As an interdisciplinary diplomat, his dedication to bridging academic insights with real-world issues drives his commitment to advancing both research and education in the field of anthropology.

**Mahfuza Rifat** is a Public Health Expert with extensive engagement in tuberculosis, health system, and health financing. Rifat is the Country Representative of International NGO Damien Foundation in Bangladesh. She has represented several review committees including Stop TB Partnership's TB REACH; she is a member of the Technical Review Panel of The Global Fund organization to fight against AIDS, tuberculosis, and malaria and a scientific reviewer of International Union Against Tuberculosis and Lung Diseases and The Health Systems Research symposiums.

**Shahaduz Zaman** has an interdisciplinary background with degrees in medical anthropology, public health, and medicine. He has more than 15 years of experience in conducting research and teaching in global public health. His research interests include hospital ethnography; socio-cultural aspects of communicable and non-communicable diseases; death dying and end of life; refugee health; role of art in health interventions, health policy, and health systems in low-income countries; and medical history.

# Preface

Tuberculosis (TB) continues to hurt us. Globally this ancient disease caused 1.3 million deaths in 2022. In the same year, an estimated 10.6 million people fell ill and started suffering as human beings have suffered for thousands upon thousands of years when their bodies become the host of the causative bacteria. Over 400,000 of these cases showed resistance to the common front-line drugs, intensifying the suffering.

Each individual does not necessarily suffer in isolation. They are marriage partners, parents, children, close and distant relatives in nuclear and extended families, friends, and colleagues. As witnesses, they share in the pain, while being aware that they may be at risk of contracting TB. Sometimes, however, people suffer alone. They may be stigmatized, excluded, or inadvertently lost in a society that is unable to offer the necessary solace and care. Inequality applies to TB as much as anything else in this profoundly stratified world, which still struggles to adequately define health and appreciate its worth.

TB continues to cost us. If we are unmoved by the suffering, the bald figures ought to bring us up short. Recent modelling suggests that not meeting the Sustainable Development Goal of reducing TB deaths by 90% by 2030 will continue to burden household and government budgets, limit economic productivity, and reduce the potential of the workforce. If TB deaths fall by only 2% (the current annual decrease) from 2020 to 2050, the economic cost will be US$17.5 trillion (95% uncertainly interval 14.9–20.4 trillion) over this period.[1]

Understanding why this disease remains so profoundly distressing and expensive is difficult and vital. It requires a breadth of approaches that can subtly and comprehensively cover the contemporary scene and integrate the disparate pasts of such an influential communicable disease. It needs a commitment to listen to others and lean into the way they think, as there is much to learn and much benefit to be gained from such an approach.

The editors and contributors to this volume have started from this premise and sought to bring their knowledge and ways of working to understanding TB. They are refreshingly largely located in the global south and all have worked there, engaging with local people as much as possible. They are aware of what this diversity of approach brings even without feeling the need to move beyond familiar tropes and boundaries in both intellectual and social terms. Equally refreshingly they don't claim to have all the answers but share their work in a spirit of collaboration. I can only recommend that readers around the world engage in a like-minded way for TB is a problem for all, not just those who suffer. It speaks for communicable diseases as an open-ended global problem that we must continue to manage with compassion and innovation, even when we cannot solve it.

Helen Bynum
Author of Spitting Blood: A History of Tuberculosis

## Note

1 Silva S, Arinaminpathy N, Atun R, Goosby E, Reid M. Economic Impact of Tuberculosis Mortality in 120 Countries and the Cost of Not Achieving the Sustainable Development Goals Tuberculosis Targets: A Full-Income Analysis. *Lancet Glob Health.* 2021 Oct;9(10):e1372–e1379. doi:10.1016/S2214-109X(21)00299-0. Epub 2021 Sep 3. Erratum in: *Lancet Glob Health.* 2021 Nov;9(11):e1507. doi:10.1016/S2214-109X(21)00445-9. PMID: 34487685; PMCID: PMC8415897.

# 1 Introduction

*Arnab Chakraborty, Janaka Jayawickrama,
and Yong-an Zhang*

This chapter introduces the book within the current global discourse of disease, health, and well-being and explains the aim of this book, which is to provide a historical and contemporary analysis of infectious diseases and their impact on human populations, taking tuberculosis (TB) as an example. According to the World Health Organisation, the burden of diseases – both infectious and non-communicable – shows a distinct difference between high- and low-income countries. In 2019, 87.8% of deaths in high-income countries were due to non-communicable diseases. In the same year, the low- and middle-income countries (LMIC) experienced the greater burden of infectious diseases, including TB, HIV, malaria, neglected communicable diseases, and hepatitis B. A popular Chinese proverb says, 'The superior doctor prevents sickness; the mediocre doctor attends to impending sickness; the inferior doctor treats actual sickness'. Uneven development and poverty can be identified as a major challenge of the burden of diseases in LMIC. Historical factors such as colonialism have a major influence on the challenges of infectious diseases we face today. TB, often regarded as a disease of poverty, continues to cast a long shadow over LMIC worldwide. In our exploration, we traverse epochs marked by social upheaval and geopolitical transformations, illuminating the historical pathways that have shaped the epidemiology and socio-economic impact of TB. At the heart of our inquiry lies a critical engagement with the United Nations Sustainable Development Goals, particularly the imperative of ending the TB epidemic as a health target. Within the framework of global health governance, we interrogate the efficacy of policy interventions and the socio-political dynamics that underpin efforts to combat TB on a global scale. By synthesizing insights from disciplines ranging from medical anthropology to political economy, we endeavour to construct a holistic understanding of the TB epidemic as a microcosm of broader challenges in achieving health equity and social justice. This chapter will elaborate these historical elements within the current challenges of the burden of infectious diseases. Among infectious diseases, TB is the 13th leading cause of death and the second leading after COVID-19 (above HIV/AIDS). Therefore, this book will focus on TB as a

DOI: 10.4324/9781032634647-1

case study to elaborate and explain the challenges of infectious diseases on human populations from a historical analysis. Towards the end of the chapter, the structure of the book and the logic of subsequent chapters will be explained. Since the middle of the twentieth century, most countries in Asia, Africa, Latin America, and the Middle East (or West Asia from our standing point), the WHO, and other international governing bodies created efforts to achieve a dream: a world free from diseases. This dream must be understood within a political, social, and economic history from the colonial era through the first generation experience of neo-colonialism. Throughout the Cold War, the waves of globalization, and post-Cold War, these "independent" countries have experienced various challenges to their governance and development, especially affecting the health and well-being of their populations.

During their independence, most countries were caught up in a fabricated debate. Historically there was this tremendous revival, a collectively generated social movement that brought independence to most countries. They took the immediate form of political movements, however had a content which transcended political agendas. For example, the South Asian independent movement included several fundamentals in a holistic approach to the life of the people. It was expected to lead not just political independence, but a good life and dignity for all. Mahatma Gandhi, among others, was at the centre of the movement for social transformation, which included education, agriculture, industries, infrastructure, and most importantly equitable health and well-being for all. However, the debate at that time, put simply, revolved around capitalism vs. socialism, or modernism vs. tradition. It is important to note that throughout a 500-year or more colonial education, punishment, and suffering, people in colonies were "colonized" in their minds. The ancient and traditional philosophies, theories, frameworks, and approaches to health and well-being were destroyed in most places.

The result of independence in most countries was a diverse mix of strategies and policies. The elites and professionals took charge and exercised the power of managing the transition. In South Asia, most of these elites and professionals were trained in the UK and came back with the idea of European modernity. In that, the fundamentals of the paradigm they adopted were not rooted either in the culture of the majority or the people. The three case studies examined in this book – Papua New Guinea, India, and Bangladesh – are former colonies and continue to suffer through colonial legacies. The work is positioned at the boundary between international history, and history of neo-colonial public health, and sociopolitical context of development (or underdevelopment). These fields come together in our focus on health and well-being as a space for the exchange of ideas on diseases, health, and well-being. This book focuses primarily on case studies from Papua New Guinea, India, and Bangladesh, however, suggests that debates, ideas, and interventions in the field of TB are global. This is because of shared histories, uneven development, and challenges of communicable diseases. As a result, the story takes us from Daru Island, Papua New Guinea to Bangalore (now Bengaluru) in India to communities in Bangladesh with detours to the USA to Sri Lanka to Cuba. Further, in Papua New Guinea, we meet Aluni and her family that struggle with TB due to uneven development. In India, we engage with the Indian National Tuberculosis programme, which started with much local and international excitement, however, failed due to various political, social, and economic encounters. In Bangladesh, we critically examine the success and challenges of person-centred care for TB through community engagement. We attempt to understand these individual, community, and intervention stories from a development perspective. In that, perhaps the most important shift occurred during the Cold War period was the emergence of the notion that health is a responsibility of governments and the right of citizens. This was drastically different from earlier approaches to public health in colonies in Asia and Africa. The colonial administrations mostly neglected and ignored epidemics, and at best, they were attempting to prevent or respond to diseases to ensure the productivity of labour. In 1948, the WHO constitution declared health as a fundamental human right.

Working through and with national governments, the WHO aimed to transform health and well-being of the world population. Due to various burdens of resources and political challenges, the WHO found its strength in science and technology. This took away the approaches and discussions about the socioeconomic roots, and political implications of health and well-being as well as the structures of health services. In return, the WHO developed strategies for targeted interventions as a tool of technical assistance, allowing health services to take responsibility away from communities, especially from the rural and urban poor. Starting from countless pilot projects and demonstration sites, the WHO conducted various campaigns, from Bacillus Calmette-Guérin (BCG) vaccination against TB, penicillin against infectious diseases, and DDT against malaria. As governments became responsible for delivering health and well-being, lack of resources and finances became the major problem. Although most countries attempted to provide health for all, it became impossible due to developmental challenges. Over the past 30 years, the increased presence in the private sector started to see the commercialization of health and well-being, which challenged the WHO constitution, which claimed health as a fundamental human right. Prevention of diseases became less important; however, "firefighting" diseases became important. As we started this chapter with an Asian proverb, what we see today is inferior health services treating actual sicknesses.

## Communicable Disease, Health, and Well-being

Like natural hazards, communicable diseases have been part of the human civilization from the beginning. We hear many legends about epidemic outbreaks in our shared histories in Asia, Africa, and many other places. However, until the European colonization project, communicable diseases were not treated as something to be studied and understood. Both the Liverpool School of Tropical Medicine and London School of Hygiene and Tropical Medicine were founded on the back of slave trade. At the same time, this rise of science and technology during the European colonial project undermined and ignored the fact that most countries beyond Europe had health systems, and in some cases better than the new science and technology. The Ayurveda (science of life) in India, Chinese traditional medicine, Inca medical system, Mosaic health systems, and African traditional medicine all had their knowledge on prevention and treating various diseases including communicable diseases.

In World Health Report 1995, the WHO declared that poverty was the world's deadliest disease. According to the World Bank more than 712 million people lived below the poverty line in 2022 (Aguilar et al. 2024). What is visible from this data is that the rich are getting richer, and the poor are getting poorer. However, not only the socioeconomic gaps widening between the rich and the poor, but the gaps are also widening between the poor and the poorest both within and between nations. We have seen how the COVID-19 pandemic has disproportionately affected the poor and vulnerable nations and communities during 2020 and 2023. Furthermore, communicable diseases often closely connected to poverty are on the rise. Plague, TB, and cholera are taking over populations in full force. This challenges the existing and mainstream international and national health campaigns against these communicable diseases.

The WHO defines health as a state of complete physical, mental, and social well-being (WHO 1948). Given that it was a transitioning world towards the end of European wars, weaker colonial project, emergence of North America as a world power, and beginning of the Cold War, this definition was groundbreaking. However, due to changing social, cultural, economic, political, and environmental context, evolving nature of communicable disease patterns, and the climate crisis, this definition may not be relevant to most individuals and communities across the world (Lindekens and Jayawickrama 2018). In that, we also want to understand health from our own roots. *Sushruta Samhita*, the Ayurvedic textbook of medicine and surgery (sixth century BC) has one of the oldest definitions of health, which can be understood within the contemporary world: quality sleep and rest, an adequate ratio of food intake and output, and a harmonious relationship with society and nature (Lad 2002).

Within this perspective, we define well-being from a different understanding. The WHO (1948) defines positive health as a state of well-being. A 2012 report (p. 9) states that "wellbeing exists in two dimensions, subjective and objective. It comprises an individual's experience of their life as well as a comparison of life circumstances with social norms and values". Examples of life circumstances include health, education, work, social relationships, built and natural environments, security, civic engagement and governance, housing, and work-life balance. Subjective experiences include a person's overall sense of well-being, psychological functioning, and affective states. We define well-being within this book against the traditional economic explanation of the idea, by defining well-being as the ability to live with uncertainties and dangers of life, not despite them. As Jayawickrama (2008) has said,

> Dangers and uncertainties are an inescapable dimension of life, and well-being is the competence to live with uncertainty. Unpredictability makes life fulfilling, as it is part of human nature to deal with it … a process of pragmatic engagement with uncertainty can create a sense of well-being.

From this perspective, the achievement of the highest standard of health and well-being is one of the fundamental rights of every human, regardless of religion, gender, race, political belief, or social, cultural, or economic condition.

## Why TB?

In the vast panorama of infectious diseases that have plagued humanity, TB stands out as a uniquely persistent and pervasive adversary. This book focuses on TB not only because of its profound historical and contemporary impact but also due to its illustrative value in understanding the broader dynamics of infectious diseases. While numerous pathogens have wreaked havoc on human populations, TB offers a compelling case study of the intricate interplay between disease, society, and scientific progress. TB has a storied past that spans millennia, making it one of the oldest diseases known to affect humans. Its presence has been documented in ancient skeletal remains and historical texts, indicating its significant impact across different eras and cultures. Unlike many infectious diseases that appear and recede, TB has demonstrated a remarkable ability to persist through time, adapting to various social, economic, and environmental changes. This persistence underscores the disease's complex biology and its ability to exploit human vulnerabilities, making it a subject worthy of focused scholarly attention.

The choice to concentrate on TB is further justified by its dual role as both a medical and a social disease. TB has not only challenged the medical community with its elusive and adaptable nature but also shaped and been shaped by societal responses. The stigmatization of TB patients, the socioeconomic factors contributing to its spread, and the public health policies developed in response to outbreaks reveal much about the interplay between health and society. Studying TB provides insights into the ways in which health disparities and social determinants influence disease dynamics and outcomes. Moreover, TB remains a critical global health issue even today. Despite the availability of effective treatments, TB continues to cause significant morbidity and mortality, particularly in LMIC. The emergence of multidrug-resistant TB and extensively drug-resistant TB poses a formidable challenge to current treatment protocols and public health strategies. By focusing on TB, this book aims to highlight the ongoing relevance of this disease and the urgent need for sustained research, policy attention, and resource allocation to combat its spread.

In addition to its historical and contemporary significance, TB serves as a paradigm for understanding infectious diseases' evolution and persistence. The pathogen's ability to develop resistance to antibiotics mirrors broader trends in microbial resistance, making TB a critical case study for the field of infectious diseases. Lessons learned from TB research and control efforts are applicable to other infectious diseases, offering valuable strategies and cautionary tales for dealing with emerging and re-emerging pathogens. The choice to focus on TB is also motivated by its illustrative power in public health innovation and response. From the establishment of early sanatoria to the development of the BCG vaccine, TB has driven significant advances in medical science and public health infrastructure. The global efforts to eradicate TB, including the WHO's End TB Strategy, exemplify international collaboration and commitment to combating a common enemy. These initiatives offer valuable lessons in the complexities of global health governance, resource allocation, and the implementation of large-scale public health interventions.

Furthermore, TB has been a silent companion to many pivotal moments in human history, from the decline of the Roman Empire to the Industrial Revolution. Its impact on the arts and literature, seen in the works of writers like Rabindranath Tagore and Gabriel Garcia Marquez, highlights the cultural significance of the disease. TB's influence on human behaviour and societal structures provides a unique lens through which to study historical and contemporary human experiences. This exploration of TB aims to provide a comprehensive overview of its history, epidemiology, and societal impact. By delving into the specifics of TB, we can better appreciate the broader challenges and triumphs in the fight against infectious diseases. Through this focused lens, we aim to contribute to the ongoing discourse on global health and the complex interrelations between pathogens, hosts, and the environment. The study of TB is not merely a study of a disease but an examination of the resilience, ingenuity, and adaptability of the human spirit in the face of enduring adversity.

## Methodological Approach

This book is interdiciplinary in nature, hence we haven't deployed any specific methodological approach. Since, it is titled, '*A Brief History of Tuberculosis*', we have a thorough historiographical literature review and analysis of existing works. Through close reading and contextual analysis, we trace the evolving understanding of TB across different historical epochs, elucidating the shifting paradigms of disease causation, prevention, and treatment. Textual sources not only provide insights into medical knowledge and practices but also reveal broader societal attitudes towards TB and its impact on human well-being. We have also used archival sources to a great extent – particularly in Chapter 4. Archives serve as invaluable repositories of historical memory, offering glimpses into the social, economic, and cultural contexts in which TB emerged and proliferated. We have also employed historiographical synthesis – drawing upon seminal works by historians, epidemiologists, and public health scholars, we interrogate prevailing narratives surrounding TB and offer fresh perspectives informed by contemporary historiographical debates. By situating our analysis within broader intellectual currents and disciplinary frameworks, we aim to enrich our understanding of TB as a complex historical phenomenon. Finally, recognizing the multidimensional nature of TB as a global health challenge, this book adopts an interdisciplinary lens that encompasses insights from fields such as history, anthropology, global health, disaster risk reduction, and human geography.

## What This Book Is About

This book is not a medical textbook. Nor this is a history book on TB or communicable diseases. The primary aim of this book is to provide a brief historical and contemporary social analysis of TB as a communicable disease. By bringing on contemporary and historical case examples, this book explores the challenges faced by practitioners, policymakers, and social science researchers in developing effective interventions to combat communicable diseases. Throughout the book, we examine various social determinants including poverty, inequality, and migration.

## Flow of the Book

This book has seven chapters including Introduction and Conclusion. We, as editors, have tried to keep the flow of these chapters logical and interdisciplinary. After Introduction, Chapter 2 explains the history of TB and its contemporary challenges. It examines the threats, hopes, and differences that the world has seen over this particular disease. Chapter 3 takes us through an ethnographic journey into the small island of Papua New Guinea and uses the lens of anthropology and human geography to understand and analyse how people have suffered because of TB in that region. Chapter 4 takes a critical approach towards India and its National Tuberculosis Programme through a historical perspective. While Chapter 5 examines the more current nature of TB control in Bangladesh. While the Indian example is of a critical nature and questions the effectiveness of DOTS and the control mechanism, the story of Bangladesh is vastly different. We hoped to tease those issues out in consecutive chapters. Chapter 6 examines the cases of Sri Lanka and Cuba, to explain how the risk of TB can be reduced through various programmes and including the local community. This provides us a framework to handle disasters and infectious diseases around the world through a combination of education, public awareness, and community-based health interventions. The final chapter, Conclusion sums up the whole book project and gives some pointers for future research and potential areas that can be examined in the future.

## The Beginning of Collaborations

This book is an outcome of a thematic research on diseases, health, and well-being organized between the Research Centre for Health and Wellbeing and International Centre for Drug Policy Studies at Shanghai University. The aim of this thematic research was to critically examine the key concepts of diseases, health, and well-being beyond the dominant epistemological perspectives. In that, this research engaged with like-minded scholars from all over the world. In a changing world, it was an exciting experience to engage with different epistemological perspectives – suddenly the world opened up for analysis beyond the linear analysis of Western science.

The editors – Arnab Chakraborty, Janaka Jayawickrama, and Yong-an Zhang, come from varied backgrounds. Arnab is a medical historian; Janaka is a social anthropologist; and Yong-an is a health historian. Our diverse backgrounds, however, brought us together to critically engage with diseases, health, and well-being from a social perspective. Growing up in India, Sri Lanka, and China, respectively, and working in different contexts, we arrived at an understanding that health and well-being are located within social, political, cultural, economic, and environmental contexts. Being in the Global South has its own disadvantages, but there are many advantages.[1] One among many is that we can collaborate with everyone – regardless of their nationalities, religions, qualifications, gender, class, and backgrounds. This provided us the intellectual freedom to collaborate with people who share common attitudes and values.

Niels Brimnes is professor of history at Aarhus University in Denmark. He is a historian specializing in the history of colonialism and the history of global health, most often based on cases related to India and South Asia. He has conducted extensive research on TB in the context of India. Paul H. Mason is an Australian anthropologist with a diverse research portfolio spanning multiple continents. His fieldwork has seen him immersed in vibrant arts communities in Indonesia and Brazil, documenting rituals among religious minorities in India and Brazil, and engaging with TB patients in Vietnam and Papua New Guinea. Paul's research extends to the social, economic, and political dimensions of TB, with publications on ethics, gender, mental health, and social models of TB. Shahaduz Zaman is professor of medical anthropology and global health at Brighton Sussex Medical School in the UK. Born and bred in Bangladesh, Zaman has conducted numerous research, education, and intervention projects in the social, cultural, economic, and environmental context of Bangladesh.

Combining the disciplines of history, anthropology, global health, disaster risk reduction, and human geography was not an easy task. In a world where everyone is striving to establish interdisciplinarity and multidisciplinarity, we started from understanding each other. Niels rich experiences in conducting fieldwork in India as a young European, Paul's sense of humour and willingness to learn from everyone, Zaman's capabilities in music and creative writing have enriched the experiences as well as this book.

As editors, we have not strictly kept to a universal format for chapters. Each chapter brings the distinctiveness of the author's discipline, background, and experiences. The editing of this book comes in the form of content, concepts, arguments, and ideas.

## Note

1 Keeping in line with the South Commission Report – the Challenges to the South (1990), we use the term Global South to refer to countries that are struggling through coloniality that affect the social, political, cultural, economic, and environmental challenges to their development. Inaugurated by the 1955 Bandung Summit in Indonesia by the newly independent countries from the European colonial project, the Global South is not a geographical location, it is an idea. For details, see South Commission, *The Challenges to the South: The South Commission Report* (Geneva: South Commission, 1990).

## References

Aguilar, R.A., Diaz-Bonilla, C., Fujs, T., Lakner, C., Nguyen, M.C., Viveros, M. and Baah, S.K. (2024) March 2024 Global Poverty Update from the World Bank: First Estimates of Global Poverty until 2022 from Survey Data. Available at: https://blogs.worldbank.org/en/opendata/march-2024-global-poverty-update-from-the-world-bank--first-esti, accessed on May 16, 2024.

Jayawickrama, J. (2008) *Why Is There More Laughter in Refugee Camps than on the Streets of London?: Mental Health and Wellbeing Amongst Disaster and Development Affected Communities*, Session on mental well-being and happiness. Annual International Conference of the Royal Geographical Society/Institute for British Geographers. United Kingdom.

Lad, V. (2002) *Textbook of Ayurveda: Fundamental Principles of Ayurveda*. Albuquerque, NM: Ayurvedic Press.

Lindekens, J. and Jayawickrama, J. (2019) Where is the care in care? A polemic on medicalisation of health and humanitarianism. *Interdisciplinary Journal of Partnership Studies*, 6(2), 1–17.

World Health Organization. (1948) *Definition of Health*. Available at: https://www.who.int/suggestions/faq/zh/index.html, accessed on May 16, 2024. https://www.who.int/about/governance/constitution.

World Health Organisation. (1995) *World Health Report 1995: Bridging Gaps, Fostering Development*. Geneva: WHO.

# 2 History of tuberculosis and contemporary challenges

*Arnab Chakraborty and Janaka Jayawickrama*

## Introduction

"There have been as many plagues as wars in history, yet always plagues and wars take people equally by surprise" – a quote from the novel "La Peste" by Albert Camus was used by World Health Organisation (WHO) Director-General Tedros Adhanom Ghebreyesus to mark four years of the COVID-19 pandemic. While this is true for most diseases, the case of tuberculosis (TB) is vastly different. Throughout human history, TB has always captured the imagination of writers around the world, and this statement holds across centuries. From Fyodor Dostoyevsky and Leo Tolstoy to Thomas Mann and Rabindranath Tagore have incorporated the ravages of this disease. From Mann's Nobel Prize-winning novel, *The Magic Mountain* to greatest films such as *Pather Panchali* by Satyajit Ray, TB was well known as the biggest killer of the nineteenth century. The prospect of a disease that can be casually contracted while walking the streets or talking to friends/strangers was eerily familiar with the diseases that were fought and presumably won in the early twentieth century. But, was it really the case? So, while looking through history and trying to understand the impact of TB in historical terms, it is essential to understand how TB as a disease was so impactful, it was a known disease to most, so we had the time to prepare for it, but it has gone through stages of importance and neglience. Currently, TB is going through a state of neglect even though its impact remains severe in many parts of the world. The WHO estimated 10.4 million individuals had TB, however, only about six million cases have been reported according to the 2013 report. According to the WHO Global TB Report 2020, ten million people were newly diagnosed with TB in 2019. TB is preventable, at least that is what the global experts believed. The highest incidence of TB cases has occurred in the Southeast Asian region, with 44% of cases, followed by the African continent (25%) and the Western Pacific (18%). The COVID-19 pandemic has crippled most of the existing systems of detection, treatment, prevention, and diagnosis of TB and most other infectious diseases (Ryckman, 2023). It will take a few years to truly understand the full impact of the pandemic on TB and other infectious diseases, so the health policymakers should

DOI: 10.4324/9781032634647-2

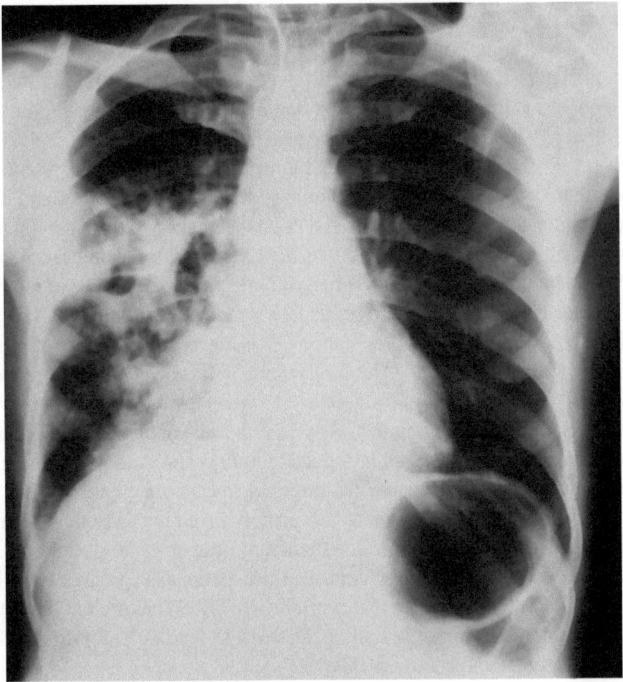

*Figure 2.1* Pulmonary TB: plain chest x-ray photo

start preparing, rebuilding, and reconstructing the healthcare infrastructure in the post-coronial world. If we look at the WHO data post-pandemic, it certainly seems like TB, in particular, should receive more attention from health organizations and funders to eliminate or at the very least reduce the burden, particularly from the developing countries. COVID-related disruptions are estimated to have resulted in almost half a million excess deaths in the three-year period of 2020–2022 (Global Tuberculosis Report 2023, WHO). TB remained the second leading cause of death from a single infectious agent in 2022, only after COVID-19 (Global Tuberculosis Report 2023, WHO) (Figure 2.1).

The big question that this chapter and subsequently this book asks is, were we ever close to beating the disease or did the global focus shift to newer diseases? This chapter will try to focus on these factors while examining the global history of TB. TB has remained one of the deadliest diseases to affect the living life on this planet. What is even more concerning is how long this disease has continued to haunt humans – it is estimated that TB has been around for the last 9,000 years at least. This disease has likely killed more people than any other plague – as many as one billion in the past 200 years. Although the illness may now seem like a historical footnote in high-income countries, it continues devastating poorer nations, afflicting the most disadvantaged: poor people, prisoners, and those who are HIV-positive (Moutinho 2022). All the last WHO Global TB Reports have focused on prison cases which are significantly higher, about 10 times higher than in the general population (Cords et al. 2021). About 30 years back, it was thought that infectious diseases were a problem of the past, thanks to vaccines and antibiotics, public health measures, and better socioeconomic conditions. HIV and AIDS changed everything – the devastating first example of many new infectious diseases, the latest being severe acute respiratory syndrome. At the same time, old infectious diseases have returned, and TB leads the way, particularly in its new deadly partnership with HIV and its ability to develop multidrug resistance. TB is now a leading cause of mortality in many parts of the world. The fundamental puzzle with TB is why it continues to kill about two million people a year when it can easily be cured with inexpensive, operational antibiotics. Why with the advent of multidrug-resistant disease, have no new drugs been introduced for 40 years? And why is there still no robust diagnostic test? Sputum culture and smears, tuberculin testing, and radiography are all essentially nineteenth-century inventions. Progress seems to have been lacking since effective chemotherapy was first introduced over half a century ago. How do environmental and occupational exposures contribute to the sustained high incidence and mortality of TB? What are the impacts of healthcare system weaknesses, such as inadequate funding and infrastructure, on the management and control of TB?

## TB: Still consuming the underprivileged?

TB is often referred to as a disease of poverty due to its strong association with socio-economic determinants. These determinants include poor living conditions, malnutrition, limited access to medical care, and lack of education. According to the WHO, over 95% of TB deaths occur in low- and middle-income countries (WHO 2021). This stark statistic underscores the link between economic deprivation and the prevalence of TB. Despite significant advancements in medical science and public health initiatives, TB continues to thrive in environments characterized by poverty, overcrowding, and limited access to health care. This essay explores the persistent impact of TB on underprivileged communities, examining the socio-economic factors that perpetuate its spread and the challenges in addressing this public health crisis. Living conditions play a critical role in the transmission of TB. In many underprivileged areas, individuals reside in overcrowded and poorly ventilated housing, which facilitates the spread of *Mycobacterium tuberculosis*, the bacteria causing TB. Overcrowding, combined with inadequate sanitation, creates an ideal environment for the bacteria to thrive and spread. That is why this book is exploring the complexities in the Global South, and teasing out case studies that would allow us to understand the context of TB better. These conditions are prevalent in urban slums and refugee camps, where people are forced to live in close quarters, often with limited access to clean water and proper sanitation facilities. TB is a complex disease. Unlike cholera, smallpox, and typhoid, TB has a distinct progression, presentation, and distribution. Approximately 30% of the global population has been infected with TB, but only 5%–10% will develop the disease or become infectious. This discrepancy indicates that the genetic and immunopathological factors, as well as the mechanisms by which reactivation occurs following stressors such as migration, poverty, or aging, are not fully understood (Smith et al., 2020). The primary challenge is differentiating between individuals infected with TB and those who are infectious or clinically ill. Rapid identification of cases is crucial for controlling the disease. An individual with unidentified active TB can infect an average of 10–15 people annually, highlighting the importance of cost-effective screening. Currently, sputum smears are the most reliable method, as tuberculin testing can yield false positives and negatives, and newer molecular approaches are not yet widely available. A better understanding of these complexities is essential for clinical management and controlling TB (Figure 2.2).

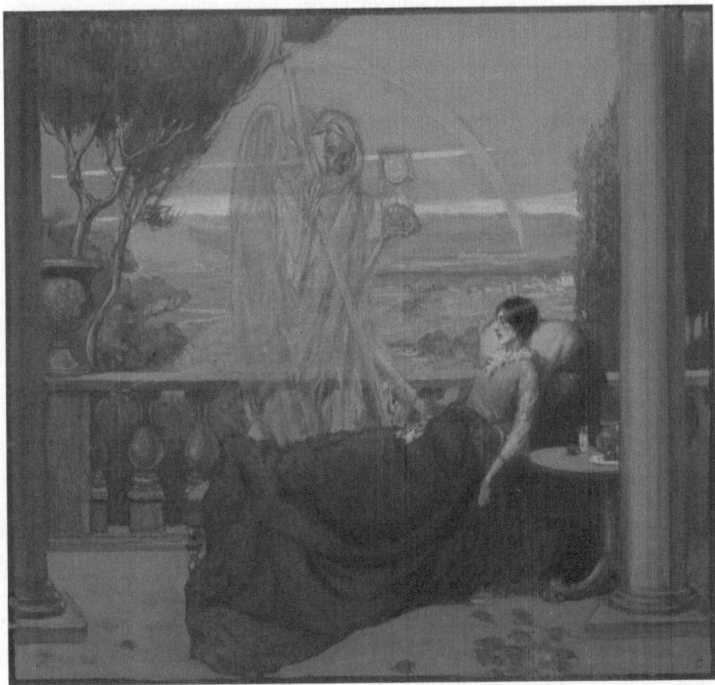

*Figure 2.2* Photo of the devastating nature of TB

Pulmonary TB, recognized as contagious by the ancient Greeks and described by Hippocrates, gained further understanding in the seventeenth century. Observations of small grey nodules in the lungs of those with consumption led to the term "tuberculosis", derived from the Latin "tuberculum", meaning a knot or nodule. The term "Phthisis" was used by the Greeks to describe the wasting away of the body associated with the disease. Despite extensive knowledge of its manifestations and progression, the etiological understanding of TB remained elusive for a long time (Brown 2018). TB is particularly insidious, causing symptoms such as night sweats, fatigue, and a persistent cough, which has historically been a hallmark of the disease. However, it has not received the attention it deserves, particularly regarding treatment. S. Lyle Cummins noted in 1939 that despite a high prevalence of TB in Burma, most people were unaware of the disease's presence because it often goes unnoticed due to its insidious nature and ability to mimic relatively good health (Cummins 1939). Hugh Stott, a medical official in Kenya, pointed out in 1956 that TB is not a "headline" disease like poliomyelitis, smallpox, or plague due to its chronicity, yet a significant outbreak would cause considerable alarm (Stott 1956). TB kills slowly, unlike the dramatic effects of plague or cholera, and lacks the disfigurement caused by polio, leading to varied levels of public concern and response.

TB is less easily transmitted than the flu or common cold, spreading through tiny airborne droplets. It thrives in poorly ventilated environments such as homeless shelters, overcrowded clinics, and prisons, and even in hospitals designed without TB control in mind (Miller et al. 2022). Primarily a disease of the poor, TB disproportionately affects certain populations. It occurs 14 times more frequently among Black individuals than White individuals and is more prevalent in large cities. People with HIV are particularly vulnerable, with up to 40% of AIDS patients having active TB, which progresses more rapidly due to their weakened immune systems. Although treatable with proper medical care and drugs, the proportion of drug-resistant TB strains has more than doubled in the last decade. The WHO declared a 'Global Tuberculosis Emergency' in 1993 due to the increasing number of TB cases worldwide, following a decline in interest during the 1970s (WHO 1993). This resurgence was partly due to an outbreak of drug-resistant TB in New York City prisons and hospitals in 1991, highlighting that TB had never disappeared from vulnerable populations (Gandy and Zumla, 2016; Koch, 2013). This period saw health experts raising alarms about increasing TB rates and the spread of multidrug-resistant tuberculosis (MDR-TB) (Koch 2018). The fact that TB affects some populations more than others is concerning. An article in the Boston Medical and Surgical Journal noted that TB was unknown among North American Indians and less common in rural areas than in cities. It also suggested that the disease was linked to lifestyle factors such as sedentary habits and intemperance, affecting women more than men due to their less physically demanding work (Rush, 1815).

Educational disparities also contribute to the burden of TB among the underprivileged. Lack of education can result in poor awareness about TB, its symptoms, and the importance of seeking early medical intervention. Misconceptions and stigma surrounding TB further hinder efforts to control its spread. In many communities, TB is associated with social stigma, leading to delays in seeking treatment and reluctance to disclose the disease. Education and community engagement are essential in dispelling myths and reducing the stigma associated with TB. Controlling TB in underprivileged populations presents numerous challenges. One major challenge is the development and spread of MDR-TB. MDR-TB arises when the bacteria become resistant to the most effective anti-TB drugs, typically due to incomplete or inadequate treatment. The WHO reports that MDR-TB is a growing concern, particularly in countries with weak healthcare systems (WHO 2021). Treating MDR-TB is more complex, requiring longer treatment durations and more expensive medications, which are often out of reach for the underprivileged.

## TB: A global scourge in the recent past

In the nineteenth century, TB was primarily managed through institutional treatments in sanatoria, which were accessible mainly to affluent populations. Despite the limited direct impact of these interventions, TB incidence in Europe and North America declined due to overall improvements in living conditions. The mid-twentieth century ushered in a new era with the advent of the BCG vaccine and antibiotic therapies, shifting the focus to developing countries. During this period, mass vaccination campaigns and clinical trials dominated TB control efforts, largely coordinated by the WHO. By the 1960s, many nations in the Global South implemented national TB control programs, integrating new biomedical technologies into broader health services. However, a perceived decline in TB's threat led to reduced international focus until the 1990s, when the HIV epidemic and outbreaks of MDR-TB sparked renewed interest. By the mid-1990s, the US media was alarmed by the statistical data indicating a health crisis, and the former Soviet Union became a source of concern for spreading MDR-TB. This situation eventually led to the development of new geographies of blame and the segregation of people based on diseases and their domicile (Koch, 2013).

Emily Abel highlights the significant role of the politics of exclusion of the immigrant population in the spread of TB in the UK (Abel 2007). Low-income TB sufferers responded to public health programs in various ways. Once services became available, some patients sought clinic care, followed medical recommendations, and accepted placement in hospitals and sanatoriums. However, many others disregarded clinic appointments, rejected advice, and either did not enrol in institutions or left soon after arrival. The exclusionary campaign elicited diverse reactions; while some Mexicans, Filipinos, and "inter-state migrants" welcomed the opportunity to leave Los Angeles during the 1930s, most resisted expulsion. Certain groups and individuals challenged prevailing assumptions about who should be considered a burden and who a resource, asserting their right to remain in the city and share equally in its social and economic benefits (Abel 2007). In many developing nations across the Global South, TB remains a pervasive threat, taking a heavy toll on individuals, families, and entire communities. For example, in Nigeria, TB is a significant public health concern and economic burden. Despite efforts to expand access to treatment through the National TB Control Program, challenges such as inadequate healthcare infrastructure, limited diagnostic capacity, and social stigma persist, hindering progress in TB control. Moreover, the emergence of drug-resistant TB strains presents a formidable challenge, with the cost and complexity of treatment placing additional strain on already overburdened health systems (WHO 2021).

Similarly, in South Africa, TB is closely linked to the HIV/AIDS epidemic, with some of the highest co-infection rates globally. The legacy of apartheid, characterized by entrenched inequalities and disparities in healthcare access, exacerbates the TB epidemic, particularly in urban townships and informal settlements. Despite significant investments in TB control efforts, including the provision of free TB treatment through the public health system, challenges such as poor treatment adherence, delayed diagnosis, and inadequate infection control persist, fuelling the spread of the disease.

Nigeria ranks among the top TB burden countries globally, with a high incidence of both pulmonary and extrapulmonary TB. The country's large population, high prevalence of HIV, and inadequate healthcare infrastructure contribute to the persistence of TB. Nigeria faces challenges in TB diagnosis, including limited access to TB diagnostic facilities, delays in specimen transportation, and insufficient laboratory capacity. These challenges hinder early detection and treatment initiation, leading to poor treatment outcomes. HIV/TB co-infection is a significant challenge in Nigeria, particularly in urban areas with high HIV prevalence. The intersection of TB and HIV epidemics poses complex clinical management challenges and underscores the importance of integrated TB/HIV services.

The Philippines ranks among the high TB burden countries in the Western Pacific Region, with a high incidence of both drug-susceptible and drug-resistant TB. Overcrowded urban areas, poverty, and limited access to healthcare services contribute to the persistence of TB in the Philippines. The Philippines has implemented various strategies to control TB, including strengthening TB diagnostic and treatment services, expanding access to TB medications, and promoting community-based TB care. However, challenges such as limited healthcare infrastructure and funding constraints continue to impede TB control efforts (Department of Health Philippines 2020, https://doh.gov.ph). Thailand has made significant progress in TB control over the years, with declining TB incidence rates. However, TB remains a public health concern, particularly among marginalized populations such as migrant workers and people living in urban slums. Thailand's TB control efforts include comprehensive TB screening and treatment programmes, public awareness campaigns, and strengthening of TB surveillance systems. Collaborative efforts between government agencies, non-governmental organizations, and international partners have contributed to the success of TB control initiatives in Thailand.

In India, TB remains a leading cause of morbidity and mortality, disproportionately affecting marginalized populations such as urban slum dwellers, migrant workers, and indigenous communities. The country's vast and diverse landscape presents unique challenges to TB control, with variations in epidemiology, healthcare infrastructure, and cultural practices influencing the distribution and burden of the disease. Efforts to combat TB in India have been hampered by factors such as poverty, overcrowding, and limited access to health care in rural and remote areas. However, innovative approaches such as the use of mobile health technologies and community-based interventions hold promise for improving TB detection, treatment, and adherence in resource-constrained settings (Rao 2006).

In Brazil, TB is not only a public health challenge but also a social justice issue, with marginalized populations such as indigenous communities, urban poor, and prisoners bearing a disproportionate burden of the disease. The country's decentralized healthcare system, while providing universal access to TB diagnosis and treatment, faces challenges such as fragmented care, inequitable resource distribution, and gaps in surveillance and monitoring. Additionally, socio-economic factors such as income inequality, urbanization, and migration contribute to the persistence of TB in vulnerable communities, highlighting the need for comprehensive, rights-based approaches to TB control that address underlying social determinants of health.

These examples illustrate the complex interplay between TB and socio-economic factors in developing nations, underscoring the importance of context-specific interventions that address the root causes of the disease. From strengthening health systems and expanding access to diagnostic tools and treatment to addressing social determinants of health and promoting community engagement, a multi-sectoral approach is essential to overcoming the challenges posed by TB in the Global South. By prioritizing equity, solidarity, and human rights in TB control efforts, we can work towards a future where TB is no longer a threat to global health security, and all individuals have the opportunity to lead healthy and productive lives.

Evidence of its antiquity comes from many parts of the world, including mummified remains in Egypt, gravesites in Europe, and skeletons in the New World. It almost certainly originated in Africa, likely in the east, and spread globally as humans migrated approximately seventy thousand years ago. It further expanded during the Neolithic Demographic Transition, a period of significant human population growth, settlement, and early agriculture. The disease may have been evolving for three hundred million years. Although not exclusive to humans – there are bovine and other forms – it is possibly the oldest human disease. Age, intractability, and prevalence are among its essential characteristics (Bynum 2012). As Helen Bynum demonstrates in her comprehensive history of TB, the disease has been a subject of debate and contemplation for as long as people have been documenting their observations (Bynum 2012).

## An overview of TB: A short historiography

The history of TB is rich and intricate. The transformation from the term "consumption" – a vague, debilitating condition marked by wasting and weakness – to "tuberculosis" occurred when the disease was identified as a specific infectious condition caused by the tubercle bacilli. This identification only became possible with Robert Koch's discovery in 1882. The transition was not immediate, as previous conceptions of the disease persisted. However, by the early twentieth century, the understanding of TB as an infectious disease transmitted among humans was well established. Since then, efforts to control TB have focused on either eliminating the bacillus from the body or preventing infection in the first place (Daniel 2000).

Historically, many have analysed the decline of TB in certain regions while it remains prevalent in others. As a historian, it is essential to consider various factors that contribute to the decline of TB, such as improved living standards, including adequate nutrition and housing, access to medical advancements like antibiotics, and supportive health and social policies. These factors collectively reduce infection risk, subsequently decreasing TB incidence. Conversely, TB persists in areas with limited access to drugs and where conditions like poor housing, malnutrition, and comorbidities such as HIV/AIDS are prevalent. The complexity of TB necessitates multiple explanations for its varying prevalence across different regions. It is also crucial to avoid the simplistic notion that biomedical approaches are ineffective or that underprivileged regions should rely solely on "appropriate technology" rather than benefiting from medical advancements. Eradicating poverty would significantly reduce TB, but since this is not an immediate possibility, advances in biotechnology, including new vaccines, shorter antibiotic regimens, and improved diagnostic tools, remain critical and urgently needed (Feldberg 1995).

Georgina Feldberg (1995) highlighted that early nineteenth-century concerns about consumption persisted well into the late 1800s as TB continued to be a leading cause of death in the USA. The decline in death rates post-1850 could be attributed to various factors, including evolving disease definitions, improved record-keeping, or genuine mortality reduction, with recorded deaths decreasing by nearly a third from 1850 to 1890. Dr. Lawrence F. Flick (1925), a pioneer in TB prevention, encapsulated the historical understanding of TB in his work "Development of Our Knowledge of Tuberculosis", emphasizing the significance of comprehending the disease's history to pave the way for its eradication. Similarly, S. Lyle Cummins (1949) in "Tuberculosis in History", celebrated Robert Koch's discovery as a monumental breakthrough, marking a definitive turning point in TB history. Selman Waksman (1964), credited with isolating streptomycin, underscored the post-1943 advancements in chemotherapy as pivotal in the fight against TB. W.A. Murray's (1981) autobiographical account, "A Life Worth Living", reflects on his personal contributions to TB control during a period of significant medical advancements. George Jasper Wherret's (1977) "The Miracle of Empty Beds" and Thomas Daniel's (2000) "Pioneers in Medicine and Their Impact on Tuberculosis" further illustrate the genre of TB historiography. Daniel's work profiles six key figures whose contributions spanned pathology, bacteriology, public health, immunology, epidemiology, and antibiotics, highlighting the transition of medicine into an evidence-based discipline. Burnham (2005) noted that traditional medical history often served to establish an identity among doctors, a theme evident in the works of the authors mentioned. Daniel's motivation stemmed from his extensive involvement in chest diseases, aiming to educate current and future medical professionals about their intellectual heritage to inspire further scientific breakthroughs.

Various historians have approached the study of TB from different perspectives. Henry Sigerist, from Johns Hopkins University, briefly referred to TB as "an extremely social disease", without further elaboration (Sigerist 1936). René and Jean Dubos (1952) expanded on this, describing TB as a social disease whose severity stemmed from societal flaws and individual behaviours. Despite recognizing the social dimensions of TB, they maintained a progressive view, suggesting that once the cause of TB was identified, preventive measures became apparent and logical (Dubos and Dubos 1952).

The critical examination of modern medicine intensified in the 1970s, significantly influenced by Ivan Illich. In his book "Limits to Medicine", Illich (1976) criticized the medical establishment as a major health threat, citing physician-caused illnesses (iatrogenesis) and the broader medicalization of life. His examples of clinical iatrogenesis, many derived from René Dubos's works, included the emergence of antibiotic-resistant bacteria – a problem in TB treatment since streptomycin's introduction. This critique spurred new historical approaches to medicine, including TB (Illich 1976). Susan Sontag's "Illness as Metaphor" (1978) was a pivotal work in this new wave, exploring the varied meanings of disease experiences. Her reliance on Dubos's history underscored the cultural and individual interpretations of TB (Sontag 1978). Thomas McKeown, a social medicine professor at Birmingham University, profoundly influenced this new social history of medicine. His research argued that improvements in living standards, rather than medical advancements, primarily drove mortality declines, a thesis central to his books "The Modern Rise of Population" and "The Role of Medicine" (McKeown 1979). McKeown demonstrated that TB mortality rates in Britain had significantly decreased before the advent of modern treatments, challenging the medical profession's claims to historical prestige (McKeown 1970).

In 1970, McKeown emphasized the need for the social history of medicine to prioritize public interest (McKeown 1970). Charles Webster, a later president of the Society for the Social History of Medicine (SSHM), advocated for a shift away from linear medical progress narratives towards understanding societal dynamics (Webster 1976). By 1980, Samuel Shortt acknowledged the rise of the "new social history of medicine", essential to understanding social history itself (Shortt, 1983). The 1980s saw social historians focusing on TB. Nancy Tomes, reviewing TB histories in 1989, noted a renaissance of scholarly interest, driven by the social construction of illness and the interplay of biological and cultural realities (Tomes 1989). This revival continued, with numerous monographs and articles examining national case studies and public health policies in countries such as Sweden, Britain, France, Germany, Canada, South Africa, Japan, and Austria. These studies highlighted the diverse experiences and constructions of TB across different contexts (Tomes 1989). The escalation of TB cases due to the HIV/AIDS pandemic prompted the WHO to declare TB a global emergency in 1993, emphasizing the threat of drug-resistant strains (WHO 1993).

Linda Bryder (1988) provided a comprehensive social history of TB in modern Britain, while David Barnes (1995) examined TB in France. The resurgence of TB in the West spurred further historical interest, with scholars like Bates (1992), Sheila Rothman, Georgina Feldberg, and Katherine Ott exploring TB's history in North America. Bates analysed patient correspondence with Dr. Lawrence Flick, a TB sufferer himself, while Rothman used personal diaries and letters from over a hundred sufferers to weave a social history of TB in America, encompassing familial, professional, and spiritual dimensions (Rothman 1995). Japanese scholars also contributed to TB historiography, with notable works by Johnston (1995). Flurin Condrau and Elisabeth Dietrich-Daum examined German experiences of TB in the early 2000s, while Anne Hardy provided a comprehensive view of TB in the West (Condrau 2000; Hardy 2003; Dietrich-Daum 2007). Matthew Gandy and Alimuddin Zumla described TB's history as marked by medical failures, reinforcing the urgency of addressing the disease's resurgence (Gandy and Zumla 2003). In non-Western contexts, scholars like Mark Harrison, Michael Worboys, and B. Eswara Rao explored TB in British India and the Madras Presidency, respectively (Harrison and Worboys 1997; Rao 2006). Bridie Andrews and Margaret Jones studied TB in China and Hong Kong, and Laurence Monnais and Aaron Moralina researched TB control in Vietnam and the Philippines, respectively (Andrews 1997; Monnais 2006; Moralina 2009).

Historians have delved into the experiences of "ordinary" TB sufferers, aiming to capture the multifaceted impact of the disease on individuals and communities. Sheila Rothman's meticulous examination of personal diaries and letters from over a hundred TB sufferers in America offered insights into the social dimensions of TB (Rothman 1995). While such efforts shed light on various aspects of TB's influence, historians like Rothman faced challenges in ensuring broad representativeness among their subjects. Rothman acknowledged the exceptional status of individuals like Deborah Fiske, a wealthy and educated woman whose experiences might not reflect those of typical TB sufferers. Despite this, Rothman contended that Fiske's life illustrated the pervasive effects of TB on education, marriage, child-rearing, friendships, religious beliefs, and interactions with medical professionals, asserting that these experiences epitomized the broader community's struggles with the disease (Rothman 1995).

Erving Goffman's "total institution" theory provided a theoretical framework for understanding this phenomenon, highlighting the transformative impact of the sanatorium experience on patients' lives (Goffman 1961).

Historical analyses of doctor-patient relationships within and outside sanatoria challenged the notion of patients as passive recipients of medical care. Scholars argued that patients actively negotiated treatment and care, shaping their healthcare experiences (Lerner, 1996). Barron Lerner's study of Firland Sanatorium, Seattle, illustrated the complex dynamics between staff and patients, revealing instances of negotiation and bargaining despite apparent coercive measures (Lerner, 1996). Moreover, historians like Katherine Ott highlighted the evolution of TB treatment paradigms, from nineteenth-century constitutional affliction perspectives to twentieth-century technologically driven approaches (Ott, 1996). Ott and others critiqued contemporary TB control strategies, emphasizing the need for greater consideration of patients' social contexts and experiences (Ott, 1996). Rothman emphasized the profound impact of disease policies on individual lives, advocating for a person-centred approach to disease history (Rothman 1995).

In addressing TB's modern challenges, researchers like Randall Packard, Sunil Amrith, and Niels Brimnes explored TB's social and racial dimensions in South Africa, South and Southeast Asia, and India, respectively (Packard 1989; Amrith 2006; Brimnes 2016). Christoph Gradmann and Helen Bynum has also written on histories of TB from different perspectives (Gradmann, 2001; Bynum 2012) Global histories of TB, such as those by McMillen, provided comprehensive accounts of post-war TB control efforts, underscoring the ongoing importance of historical insights in shaping contemporary approaches to TB management (McMillen 2015). Paul Mason has also written extensively on TB from anthropological perspectives (Mason 2019) while Rachel Core has recently published a book exploring TB control in Shanghai, China (Core 2023).

## Conclusion

It is about time we get off from our internal 'Magic Mountain' and accept the severity of TB in the developing world. The historical trajectory of TB reveals a complex interplay between biological, social, and environmental factors that have shaped its prevalence and impact over millennia. Our romanticized detachment, akin to life on Thomas Mann's "Magic Mountain", must give way to a pragmatic acknowledgment of TB's enduring and pervasive threat. The narrative of TB is deeply entwined with the histories of colonialism, poverty, and uneven development, highlighting the persistent inequalities that exacerbate its burden in low- and middle-income countries. The evolution of TB from an ancient scourge to a modern public health crisis illustrates how social determinants of health, such as malnutrition, diabetes, HIV infection, and lifestyle factors like smoking and alcohol use, interact to maintain its prevalence. Understanding TB requires not just a medical or biological perspective but an integrative approach that considers the broader socioeconomic and environmental context.

In conclusion, the battle against TB is far from over, but it is one that can be won with a comprehensive and integrated approach. By addressing the social, economic, and environmental factors that underpin the disease, we can make significant strides towards ending the TB epidemic. It is time for the global community to come together, to move beyond our internal 'Magic Mountain', and to commit to a future where TB is no longer a threat to human health and development.

## References

Abel, E.K., (2007). Tuberculosis and the politics of exclusion: A history of public health and migration to Los Angeles. New Jersy: Rutgers University Press.

Amrith, S. (2006) *TB in South and Southeast Asia: A New History*. Cambridge University Press, London.

Andrews, B. (1997) Tuberculosis and modern China. In P. Weindling (Ed.), *International Health Organisations and Movements, 1918–1939*. Cambridge University Press, London.

Barnes, D.F. (1995) *The Making of A Social Disease: Tuberculosis in Nineteenth Century France*. Berkeley: University of California Press.

Bates, B. (1992) *Bargaining for Life: A Social History of Tuberculosis, 1876–1938*. Philadelphia: University of Pennsylvania Press.

Brimnes, N. (2016) *Languished Hopes: Tuberculosis, the State and International Assistance in Twentieth-century India*. Orient Blackswan.

Brown, R. (2018), Tackling bovine TB. Veterinary Record, 183: 697–698.

Bryder, L. (1988) *Below the Magic Mountain: A Social History of Tuberculosis in Twentieth-Century Britain*. Oxford University Press.

Burnham, J.C., (2005). What is Medical History?. London: Polity Press.

Bynum, H., 2012. Riding the waves: optimism and realism in the treatment of TB. The Lancet, 380(9852), pp.1465–1466.

Condrau, F., & Tanner, J. (2000). Working-class experiences, cholera and public health reform in nineteenth-century Switzerland. In S. Sheard, & H. Power (Eds.), Body and city: Histories of urban public health (pp. 109–122). Farnham: Ashgate Publishing Ltd.

Cords, O., Martinez, L., Warren, J.L., O'Marr, J.M., Walter, K.S., Cohen, T., Zheng, J., Ko, A.I., Croda, J. and Andrews, J.R., (2021). Incidence and prevalence of tuberculosis in incarcerated populations: a systematic review and meta-analysis. *The Lancet Public Health*, 6(5), pp.e300-e308.

Core, R.S. (2023) *Tuberculosis Control and Institutional Change in Shanghai, 1911–2011*. Hong Kong University Press.

Cummins, S.L. (1939). Primitive Tuberculosis., London: John Bale Medical Publications.

Cummins, S.L. (1949) *Tuberculosis in History: From the Seventeenth Century to Our Own Times*. Baillière: Tindall and Cox.

Daniel, T.M. (2000) *Pioneers in Medicine and their Impact on Tuberculosis*. University of Rochester Press.

Department of Health Philippines, (2020), 2020 National TB Report, Available at: https://ntp.doh.gov.ph/, Accessed on November 10, 2023.

Dietrich-Daum, E. (2007) Tuberculosis in Austria. In F. Condrau and M. Worboys (Eds.), *Tuberculosis Then and Now: Perspectives on the History of an Infectious Disease*. McGill-Queen's University Press.

Dubos, R. and Dubos, J. (1952) *The White Plague: Tuberculosis, Man, and Society*. Little, Brown and Company.

Dubos, R.J. and Dubos, J., (1987). The white plague: tuberculosis, man, and society. New Jersy: Rutgers University Press.

Feldberg, G.D. (1995) *Disease and Class: Tuberculosis and the Shaping of Modern North American Society*. New Brunswick: Rutgers University Press.

Flick, L.F. (1925) *Development of Our Knowledge of Tuberculosis*. Philadelphia: The Author.

Gandy, M. and Zumla, A. (2003) *The Return of the White Plague: Global Poverty and the 'New' Tuberculosis*. Verso.

Gandy, M. and Zumla, A., (2016). The resurgence of disease: social and historical perspectives on the "new" tuberculosis. In *Health Psychology* (pp. 230–242). Routledge.

Global tuberculosis report (2023). Geneva: World Health Organization; 2023. Licence: CC BY-NC-SA 3.0 IGO.

Gradmann, C., (2001). Robert Koch and the pressures of scientific research: tuberculosis and tuberculin. Medical history, 45(1), pp.1–32.

Goffman, E. (1961). Asylums: Essays on the social situations of mental patients and other inmates. Doubleday (Anchor).

Hardy, A. (2003) *Health and Medicine in Britain Since 1860*. Macmillan.

Harrison, M. and Worboys, M. (1997) *A Disease of Civilisation: Tuberculosis in Africa and Asia, 1900–1940*. In L. Marks and M. Worboys (Eds.), *Migrants, Minorities and Health: Historical and Contemporary Studies*. Studies in the Social History of Medicine. London: Routledge, pp. 93–124.

Illich, I., (1976). *Limits to medicine: Medical nemesis*. London: M. Boyars.

Johnston, W. (1995) *The Modern Epidemic: A History of Tuberculosis in Japan*. Harvard University Press.

Koch, E. (2013) *Free Market Tuberculosis*. Nashville, US: Vanderbilt University Press.

Lerner, B.H., (1996). Public Health Then and Now. American Journal of Public Health, 86(2).

Mason, P.H. (2019) Excluded from reciprocity: tuberculosis, conspicuous consumption and the medicalization of poverty. In *Understanding Tuberculosis and Its Control*. Routledge, pp. 206–220.

Maynard-Smith, L., Brown, C.S., Harris, R.J., Hodkinson, P., Tamne, S., Anderson, S.R. and Zenner, D., (2020). Air-travel related TB incident follow up–effectiveness and outcomes: a systematic review. *European Respiratory Journal*.

McKeown, T., (1970). A sociological approach to the history of medicine. Medical History, 14(4), pp. 342–351.

McKeown, T. (1979) *The Role of Medicine: Dream, Mirage, or Nemesis?* Princeton University Press.

McMillen, C.W. (2015) *Discovering Tuberculosis: A Global History, 1900 to the Present.* New Haven and London: Yale University Press.

Miller, K.D., Nogueira, L., Devasia, T., Mariotto, A.B., Yabroff, K.R., Jemal, A., Kramer, J. and Siegel, R.L., (2022). Cancer treatment and survivorship statistics, 2022. *CA: a cancer journal for clinicians, 72*(5), pp.409–436.

Monnais, L. (2006) *The Colonial Life of Pharmaceuticals: Marketing Medicines in the Dutch East Indies, Vietnam, and the Philippines.* Routledge.

Moralina, A.R. (2009) State, society, and sickness: tuberculosis control in the American philippines, 1910–1918. *Philippine Studies*, 57(2), 179–218.

Moutinho, S. (May 2022) Tuberculosis is the oldest pandemic, and poverty makes it continue. *Nature*, 18. Accessed at: https://www.nature.com/articles/d41586-022-01348-0

Murray, W. A., (1981), A Life Worth Living: 50 Years in Medicine, Self Published.

Ott, K. (1996) *Fevered Lives: Tuberculosis in American Culture Since 1870.* Cambridge, MA: Harvard University Press.

Packard, R.M. (1989) *White Plague, Black Labor.* Berkeley and Los Angeles, CA: University of California Press.

Rao, B.E. (2006) *Tuberculosis in the Madras Presidency: A Social History.* Orient Longman.

Rothman, S.M. (1995) *Living in the Shadow of Death: Tuberculosis and the Social Experience of Illness in American History.* Baltimore: Johns Hopkins University Press.

Rush, B. (1815) An inquiry into the comparative state of medicine, in Philadelphia, between the years 1760 and 1766, and the year 1809. In Benjamin Rush, Medical Inquiries and Observations, 4th ed. Philadelphia: M. Carey.

Ryckman, T. (February 2023) Ending tuberculosis in a post-COVID-19 world: a person-centred, equity-oriented approach. *The Lancet Infectitous Diseases*, 23(2), E59–E66.

Shortt, S.E., (1983). Physicians, science, and status: issues in the professionalization of Anglo-American medicine in the nineteenth century. *Medical history, 27*(1), pp. 51–68.

Sigerist, H.E. (1936) *Civilization and Disease.* Cornell University Press.

Stott, D. H., (1956), Unsettled Children and Their Families, London: University of London Press.

Sontag, S. (1978) *Illness as Metaphor.* Farrar, Straus and Giroux.

Tomes, N. (1989) The white plague and the red plague: a review of histories of tuberculosis. *Bulletin of the History of Medicine*, 63(2), 248–270.

Waksman, S.A., (1964). Autobiographic sketch. Perspectives in Biology and Medicine, 7(4), pp.377–398.

Wherrett, G.J., (1977). *The miracle of the empty beds: a history of tuberculosis in Canada.* Buffalo: University of Toronto Press.

Webster, C. (1976) The history of medicine and health: the importance of the social context. *Medical History*, 20(1), 1–21.

World Health Organization. Tuberculosis Unit. (1991) *Guidelines for Tuberculosis Treatment in Adults and Children in National Tuberculosis Programmes.* Geneva: World Health Organization.

World Health Organization (WHO). (1993) *Declaration of Tuberculosis as a Global Emergency.* WHO Press.

World Health Organisation, (2021), Tuberculosis, Available at: https://www.who.int/news-room/fact-sheets/detail/tuberculosis, Accessed on May 15, 2024.

# 3 Borderland tuberculosis

## The social, economic, and geopolitical contours of disease care and prevention on Daru Island, Papua New Guinea

*Paul H. Mason*

### An ethnography of cross-border tuberculosis healthcare seeking on Daru Island, Papua New Guinea

Nestled amidst the sago palms and the thick, humid air enveloping Daru Island, Aluni and her family live with her husband's extended family in a dwelling within the confines of an overcrowded housing settlement. The structure, a testament to resourceful craftsmanship, was cobbled together from repurposed timber, reinforced with sturdy mangrove posts and saplings. The leaking roof, a haphazard mosaic of salvaged iron and biri (palm) leaves, defiantly shielded its inhabitants from the worst of the relentless tropical sun and sporadic downpours, albeit with a tenuous resilience. Windows were a luxury unknown to this makeshift abode, yet slender beams of light defiantly infiltrated the walls and roof, tracing fleeting patterns across the interiors. In this settlement, homes huddled together shoulder to shoulder, with scarcely a yard between them, creating a labyrinthine maze of interconnected abodes.

The settlement, and the dwelling Aluni called home, experienced periodic overcrowding during mining compensation disbursements when mainland relatives flocked to the island. The flux of family members led to makeshift sleeping arrangements spilling over into the veranda and beneath the house. Housing dynamics during compensation periods reveal the intricate balance between familial ties and the practical constraints of space and resources. The ebb and flow in this community puts a strain against the borders of the settlement putting pressure on the surrounding natural environment.

In the cramped quarters of Aluni's dwelling, where barely enough space existed for a bilum bag between kin, food, and sometimes betel nut wrapped in slake lime are shared among the occupants. Red-stained teeth are the tangible mark of this communal act, symbolizing more than a mere sharing of commodities, but also the sharing of joys and hardships. As the population of Daru swells, families grapple with overcrowding and the scarcity of resources, unveiling a complex interplay between kinship obligations and the limitations imposed by finite resources. Kinship relations

DOI: 10.4324/9781032634647-3

oblige hospitality, and limited food resources are dutifully shared among kin. The harsh reality of food insecurity was felt strongest during these periods, but a shared commitment to the spirit of community is also strongly reinforced.

Malnourishment and overcrowding are severe health risk factors on Daru Island. The deficit of nutrition left its mark on Aluni's once robust yet now fragile frame. Her diet, dominated by sago, rice, and fish, was emblematic of the economic disparities that plague Daru Island. The increasing social and economic development gap between Daru and neighbouring islands within the Torres Strait Treaty, known as the Torres Strait Protected Zone, under-scored the uneven impact of political and economic forces (Busilacchi et al. 2018). Daru, the provincial capital of Western Province in Papua New Guinea, is a unique urban centre in the midst of the South Fly District's sprawling and rugged expanses (Busilacchi et al. 2018). Food insecurity and overcrowd-ing on the island are coupled with a lack of water, sanitation, and hygiene (Adepoyibi et al. 2019; Jops et al. 2022; Jops et al. 2023). In the 1990s, Daru was described as the most economically depressed region of Papua New Guinea (Arther 1992; Lawrence 1998).

Aluni's husband, drawn to Daru from the Madubawan area on the PNG mainland, was caught in the undertow of economic shifts catalysed by land dispossession. The legacy of Australian colonial history and mining activities had reshaped traditional landscapes, propelling individuals like Aluni's hus-band into precarious work and informal trade. Aluni, a Torres Strait Islander woman from one of the 14 PNG coastal villages referred to as PNG Treaty villages, carried with her a cultural identity shaped by historical negotiations and a connection to land fractured by Australian colonial influence, economic imbalances introduced by the growth and wane of foreign interests, the blurry lines between legal and illegal fishing trade, as well as black market firearm, drug, and animal trafficking.

Aluni was one of the few people in her family who had completed school. With scarce employment on the island, the certificate translated into meagre prospects. She had a hard-won understanding of her social, economic, and political circumstances. When she became sick with a persistent cough, loss of weight and night sweats, Aluni confronted not only the physical symptoms of her ailment, but also the looming stigma from the local community. Per-ceiving the inadequacies of local health care and wanting to escape the local stigma, she brainstormed how to access the best treatment. She felt that mak-ing her way to Australia would secure her the best chance of accessing ade-quate medical care. Poignantly, Aluni's journey to seek treatment in Australia was not simply about health-seeking and accessing medical care but about navigating social stigma, political borders, and economic hierarchies. Her Treaty status afforded her a path to Australia, a journey driven by desperation but demanding sacrifice. In a difficult decision, she decided to leave behind her husband, five-year-old daughter, and seven-year-old son, and the precari-ous life they led, in order to seek treatment in Australia.

It took Aluni and her husband more than a month to save up the necessary funds she needed for the voyage by boat to the Australian mainland. Her husband, not coming from a Treaty island, would not be able to go. The petrol alone was a month's worth of income. Hampered by her ailing health, as well as the emotions of leaving her husband and children behind, the day and half journey with an outboard motor was not easy. Upon arrival at the hospital in Australia, Aluni was isolated with suspected tuberculosis (TB). She felt alone and had no way of knowing beforehand that she was to end up staying for four years being treated for multidrug-resistant TB. During this time, she had no means of contacting her family to let them know her diagnosis or how her treatment was going. Even if her family or someone they knew had owned a phone, she had no money to call them nor any known number to call. Still, Aluni thought herself to be one of the lucky ones to be able to access treatment in Australia. Many people who were sick on Daru Island found their access to adequate health care constrained by geographic and geopolitical factors. Though at times, Aluni did feel trapped by a medical system that did not allow her to leave the hospital. Treatment was free but multi-drug therapy under direct observation was demanding. She escaped a few times to wander the streets, but with nowhere to go, and in fear that she would be reported to authorities, she promptly returned only to be scolded by the nursing staff who were otherwise kind and generous with her. Her attempts to escape the hospital, albeit brief, reveal a tension between the desire to move freely and the constraints imposed by medical protocols.

While Aluni was completing TB treatment in Australia, her husband on Daru Island had also succumbed to TB. He commenced treatment on Daru Island but tragically became lost to follow-up. He had travelled to the mainland for work only to pass away from the complications of his disease. His treatment had been challenging with his family reporting violent outbursts and psychotic episodes while taking one of the now-discontinued drugs for multidrug-resistant TB, cycloserine. Despite the provision of free medication, TB treatment still entails ancillary financial and personal costs (Mason 2019). For individuals like Aluni's husband, navigating the complexities of the healthcare system meant grappling with the dual role of assuming obligations as a patient with responsibilities to family. In a heartbreaking manifestation of this struggle, the immediate commitments of providing for his family seemed to have outweighed the need, or perhaps out-competed the ability, for Aluni's husband to complete treatment. The competing demands of illness, poverty, and familial responsibilities create a landscape of decision-making that can only be understood and reconciled by the afflicted. After their father's death, Aluni's children believed themselves orphans. They stayed in the family residence on Daru Island and were looked after by their paternal aunt and the extended family.

By herself in the foreign environment of the Australian hospital, Aluni felt isolated. She did not know anyone and longed to return to her family. She remained committed to completing her treatment. The pills from her complicated drug regimen often made her feel nauseous, but she found ways to stock and time her hospital meals so that she could avoid feeling nauseous. After four lonely years within the Australian hospital's TB ward, Aluni was finally released with a medical certificate giving her the all-clear. Resourcefully, she found a way to island hop home and make her way back to her family. She was not to know that her husband had become a casualty of TB not simply due to the absence of comprehensive healthcare infrastructure, but due to economic conditions that precluded him from staying near the clinic to collect his medication and follow directly observed treatment himself. In Aluni's absence, her children had been cared for by her husband's family, unaware that Aluni would ever return (Figure 3.1).

One grey and cloudy day, as Aluni's daughter, now nine years old, played along the muddy shores of Daru, a dinghy slowly emerged on the horizon. Drawing closer, it brought with it an unexpected moment of disbelief. As the vessel drew near, Aluni's daughter thought she saw a ghost. At the boat's bow stood a woman who bore a striking resemblance to her mother. Aluni, peering eagerly towards the shoreline, took a brief moment to grasp that the little girl was her own daughter. In a surge of emotion, mother and daughter exchanged glances. Recognizing each other, they both leapt into the water. Aluni's daughter had never waded out so far. Before being almost swallowed by the water's depths, Aluni gently lifted her daughter from the water. She was much, much bigger than Aluni remembered. Sorrow for the time lost

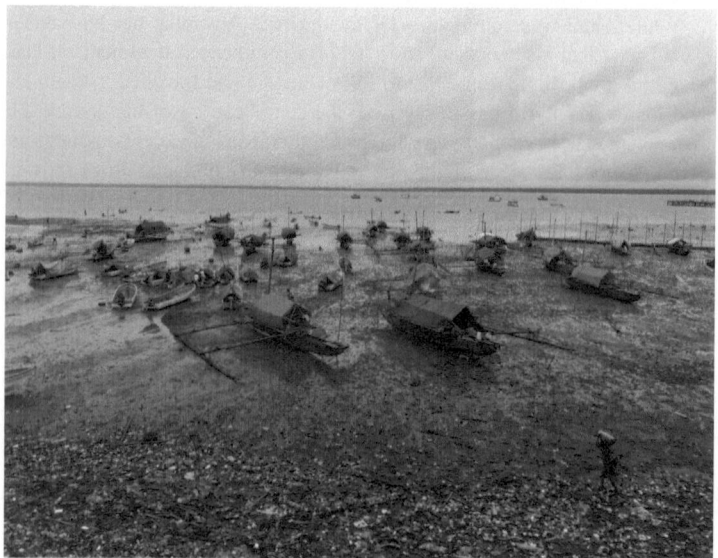

*Figure 3.1* Image of boats on the middle shoreline of Daru Island

together rippled through her trembling limbs. The pain of separation met the elation of rediscovery. The waves closed in around them as they looked into each other's tearful eyes. Sobbing, they embraced each other as more waves crashed around them. In the undulating embrace of the water, mother and daughter found solace and renewal.

The ethnographic vignette ends here with the heart-wrenching embrace between a mother who had fought against the odds and a daughter who had believed her lost. This heartbreaking moment lays bare the human cost of a disease thriving in the shadow of political and economic complexities. The human experience of TB disease goes beyond mere medical diagnosis and pharmaceutical treatment. Far from a simple health complaint, the harsh realities of TB blend medical challenges with the social, economic, and political factors that shape the disease's prevalence, dissemination across communities, and treatment outcomes for citizens. The deeply personal narratives are inseparable from the broader systemic forces at play. The impact of TB upon the lives of individuals is nuanced, multilayered, and multidimensional.

The social determinants of disease model (Simandan 2017; Maciel et al. 2018; Madjid et al. 2020) and a social construction lens (Mason et al. 2015; Dobre 2018; Hayward et al. 2018) come into focus in revealing the complex societal factors shaping Aluni and her husband's responses to and experiences with TB. Furthermore, the concept of syndemic (Mitchell et al. 2018; Zvonareva et al. 2019) adds depth to our understanding, emphasizing the intersection of TB with other social and medical issues, creating a bio-social complexity that challenges traditional models of disease management. In particular, Aluni's story is a microcosm of the broader TB riskscapes (Jops et al. 2022) in the context of cross-border healthcare seeking. Her TB treatment predates the initiation of a Provincial TB Program, established in 2014, to mitigate the impact of drug-sensitive and drug-resistant TB in Western Province. Despite the programme's implementation, PNG patients from Treaty villages continue to encounter delays in reaching Daru General Hospital for TB diagnostics and treatment. A study by Foster et al. (2022) reveals that many patients meeting evacuation criteria between 2016 and 2019 were not transported to Australia. Furthermore, patients referred back to Daru General Hospital in PNG faced their own set of challenges, including lost follow-ups and, unfortunately, mortality. The trappings of cross-border healthcare dynamics raise questions about consistency, equity, and the emergent duty of care associated with the movement of people between PNG and Australia. The findings emphasize the need for ongoing monitoring and evaluation of patient outcomes for transparency and justice in healthcare practices that extend beyond national borders.

Aluni's experiences speak to the interconnectedness of health, politics, and economy, where the management of disease is deeply embedded in socio-cultural structures. At different levels of "a four-tier system of privilege" (Chaudhry 2020), the health outcomes for Aluni, a Treaty villager, and her deceased husband, a non-Treaty villager, diverged starkly. Notably, regional evidence indicates inferior TB treatment outcomes for men, a phenomenon unexplainable in either biological or universal cultural terms (Mason et al. 2017). Aluni's experience with TB intersects with other variable factors such as her gender, cultural identity, citizenship status, socioeconomic living conditions, access to education, and the global distribution of healthcare resources. This ethnographic narrative compels us to question the sustainability of TB care and prevention if a deeper examination of the political economy and social production of TB remains absent. In Daru and beyond, TB's persistence is not exclusively a biological challenge but a problem entwining itself with historical legacies, political complexities, and the asymmetric gradients of intersecting economic structures.

The ethnographic vignette presented is a composite narrative distilled from participant-observation and semi-structured interviews conducted during a field trip to Daru Island, Papua New Guinea, in January 2018. The research approach involved working alongside TB healthcare staff in the community, allowing for deep engagement and understanding of the social, cultural, and living conditions at play. Ethical considerations, including respect for the privacy and anonymity of individuals, were paramount throughout the study. All participants were informed about the nature and purpose of the research, and their consent was obtained before any interviews or observations. To ensure anonymity, pseudonyms have been used, and identifying details have been altered or omitted. The composite nature of the case study emerges from a synthesis of various individuals' experiences, reflecting salient themes and challenges faced by TB patients in the region. This approach aims to protect the identity and dignity of the participants while providing a nuanced understanding of the broader context of TB on Daru Island.

## Precarity and the geographical imperatives of TB in the borderlands

A TB diagnosis not only signifies a medical condition but also introduces geographical imperatives, reshaping the landscape of belonging in Daru. Here, the location of TB diagnostic and treatment facilities becomes a disruptive force, affecting both proximal and distal populations in distinct ways. Travel to the clinic is in order for the TB patients. And for families living nearby, hosting a TB patient is obliged. Proximity to healthcare services can expose communities to the vulnerabilities of transmission, as sick relatives relocate to Daru Island for diagnosis and treatment, relying on kinship ties for residency and meals while potentially still infectious. Conversely, the distance from healthcare services renders people vulnerable to diagnostic delays and the challenges of sustaining a livelihood, especially if they are moving closer to TB health services without extended family on Daru. Moreover, access to different national TB programmes is dictated by citizenship status and rights, creating manoeuvrability for the few who can afford it. In the process of accepting a diagnosis or grappling with the potential consequences of denying it, or avoiding it in one location and seeking it elsewhere, personhood is redefined by TB. Personal biographies are challenged, social narratives are reshaped, and new moral imperatives are introduced.

The disruptive nature of TB extends beyond individual health to precarity, where already fragile livelihoods become more tenuous when entwined with the physical and social challenges of living with TB (Mason 2019). This intricate web of disruptions emphasizes that TB, in a broader sense, is not the sole arbiter of fate; rather, it is entwined with the structural conditions that significantly shape treatment outcomes. A critical reflection on the interplay between health, technology, and socio-political structures suggests that TB itself doesn't wield the power to end lives; instead, people, through political actions and the structures they create, become the determining factor in the fate of those affected by this disease. Put another way, TB doesn't kill people, people kill people.

The borderlands between Australia and PNG are perceived by Australian medical authorities as conduits for emerging infectious diseases (Lawrence 1998; Gilpin et al. 2008; Simpson et al. 2011; Brolan et al. 2011). Health access is not strictly a justification for travel to Australia, rather, provisions for free movement contribute to a situation where individuals from PNG, especially those grappling with TB, HIV/AIDS, cholera, dengue, or malaria, find access to Australian health services desirable and, depending upon circumstances, achievable (Brolan et al. 2011). The permeability of borderlands acts as a reminder that nation-state boundaries are multiple, shaped by practices that both construct and contest them. Humans, microbes, and pharmaceuticals traverse, navigate, and circumvent these boundaries at different speeds with varying impacts. Transborder health care, for Australians, represents a benevolent means of traversing boundaries to offer biocontainment, while also serving a self-interested strategy to fortify borders in the interest of safeguarding biosecurity and the health of national citizens. In the pre-colonial era, Australia and Papua New Guinea were not separate entities with distinct geopolitical boundaries through the Torres Strait; instead, the Torres Strait Islands were connected, not separated, by water. With the human-microbe relations of TB particularly critical in borderlands, Chuengsatiansup and Limsawart (2019) insightfully propose that TB care and prevention should transcend the prevailing biocontainment model, embracing a more flexible topological conception of spatiality that accommodates the fluid dynamics of pharmaceuticals, microbes, and human relations. Similarly, Dhavan et al. (2017) call for migrant-inclusive national TB plans, migrant-sensitive care and prevention, and the implementation of bold intersectoral policies and systems that support migrants, emphasizing the critical role of operational research.

## Biomedical disease models and the technological imperative in global TB control

Attempts to explain disease are dominated and framed by contemporary technologies, social customs, and theories of knowledge (Rosenberg 1992). How diseases are defined, understood, and treated has consequences for the lives of individuals, the making of social policy, and the organization of medical care (Rosenberg 1992; Fairchild and Oppenheimer 1998; Carel et al. 2016). Biomedical characterizations of TB typically dissociate the disease from the patient's body and lived experience. TB is often reduced to a specific type of lesion, a type of disease entity detached from its manifestation in individual patients. Consequently, therapeutic interventions are directed at the disease rather than the person. Treatments become standardized, overlooking individual variations and circumstances, as patients with the same diagnosis receive uniform treatments. The focus shifts from the subjective experiences of well-being or illness to standardized responses to treatment (Cantor 2003). Addressing the complexities of disease elimination demands a departure from reductionist approaches, necessitating the incorporation of socially oriented perspectives (Farmer 2003; Degeling et al. 2015).

Internationally standardized World Health Organisation (WHO) protocols have been politically successful in garnering funding for TB health care in various country contexts, but have insufficiently accounted for local conditions and diverse patient populations (Porter et al. 2002; Harper 2010; Koch 2013; Engel 2015; Brimnes 2016). The unintended consequences extend beyond the challenges of adapting local services to global directives; they manifest iatrogenically, contributing to the emergence of multidrug resistance (Farmer and Kim 1998; McMillen 2015). In certain regions, drug-resistant strains of TB could surpass drug-sensitive strains, potentially becoming the dominant form of the disease (Dheda and Migliori 2012; Abubakar et al. 2013; Zumla et al. 2014; Trauer et al. 2016). As WHO-mandated TB treatment programmes proliferate globally, a critical question emerges: To what extent are new patient cohorts expected to conform to these standardized approaches, and what are the implications of this standardization for diverse and context-specific health outcomes?

In the pursuit of addressing TB, the dominant biomedical model habitually attributes suboptimal treatment outcomes to inadequacies in medical technologies rather than acknowledging the intricate web of social, economic, and political infrastructures at play (Mason et al., 2020). This reliance on technological imperatives, while seemingly progressive, can inadvertently perpetuate victim-blaming narratives. The push to simplify diagnostics and treatment, under the guise of improving accessibility, implies a presumption that individuals are incapable of navigating existing technologies. This shift towards technological solutions, however well-intentioned, conveniently becomes a means of offloading responsibility and diverting attention away from addressing structural factors. The persistent emphasis on technological enhancement risks overshadowing the imperative for more profound political and economic changes essential for comprehensive health care. Consequently, this approach unwittingly perpetuates structural violence, as it maintains the very structures that deny people access to technology in the first place.

To counterbalance the prevalent technological focus within the biomedical sphere, Teo et al. (2023) propose a multifaceted approach to TB control. They emphasize the importance of social protections, advocating for measures such as income replacement and financial grants to reduce TB incidence and mortality. Additionally, the provision of health equity funds to support the economically disadvantaged is highlighted as a critical step towards improving access to healthcare services. Teo et al. further champion community-based programmes for active TB case finding, specifically targeting the most vulnerable individuals in high-burden settings. Their recommendation extends to the adoption of age-friendly healthcare principles, promoting person-centred approaches to treatment monitoring and support for enhanced treatment adherence. Recognizing the enduring physical and mental health impacts of TB, the authors stress the necessity of post-TB health and rehabilitation services. In doing so, they present a comprehensive strategy that transcends technological solutions, addressing social, economic, and healthcare system aspects for a more holistic approach to TB management.

A myopic focus on biomedical technology neglects the complex interplay of social determinants, limiting our understanding of disease to a narrow perspective. Exclusive reliance on biomedical approaches not only disregards the social realities that foster the spread of TB but also hinders the development of holistic strategies for TB prevention. Confronting the socio-economic factors driving TB prevalence and embracing the cultural nuances that shape individuals' responses to TB are key to building a successful multifactorial approach to disease prevention. By broadening our analytical scope to encompass the diverse dimensions of TB – embracing both the biological and the social – we can move beyond reductionist tendencies and pave the way for more equitable, culturally sensitive, and effective interventions. A more encompassing examination, one that incorporates the lived experiences of communities affected by TB, the economic disparities influencing healthcare access, and the political determinants shaping healthcare policies, is indispensable for constructing a truly comprehensive understanding of this global health challenge. After all, contemplating TB solely through the lens of biomedical technology, without considering the broader social, economic, and political conditions influencing its spread and control, raises a pivotal question: What will we truly know of a disease if only the disease we know?

## Global TB landscape: Beyond individual narratives

Aluni's story is one of over ten million TB narratives that unfold globally each year (Litvinjenko et al. 2023). Panning out from Aluni's story and our theoretical exploration of TB, we can think about not just the proportion of active cases that go untreated each year but also the silent presence of latent TB infections in over 1.7 billion people worldwide (Houben and Dodd 2016). These latent cases, predominantly in low- and middle-income countries, constitute a latent biological reservoir that lies dormant until triggered by malnutrition or other socio-environmental factors. Stories and experiences similar to that of Aluni isn't very difficult to find in most countries of the Global South and what this volume is trying to explore in greater detail.

Expanding our gaze from Aluni's singular journey to encompass the broader scope of the global history of TB, we encounter a narrative rich in diversity and complexity. Herein lies the significance of her story within the context of this book dedicated to unravelling this intricate history. By delving into the lived experiences of individuals like Aluni, we gain valuable insights into the cultural, social, and economic dimensions of TB across time and space. Such narratives serve as vital threads, weaving together the fabric of a holistic understanding of TB – from its ancient origins to its modern-day manifestations. Aluni's narrative finds its rightful place among the myriad voices clamouring to be heard. Her story serves as a poignant reminder of the human toll exacted by this persistent scourge, while also shedding light on the broader societal forces at play. In this way, Aluni's story becomes not only a chapter in the annals of TB history but also a beacon guiding our collective quest for understanding, empathy, and ultimately and hopefully, eradication.

People with latent TB infection carry TB mycobacterium but are asymptomatic. They have been exposed to *Mycobacterium tuberculosis* and infected but are not yet sick. Contacts of TB patients have a higher risk than the general population of becoming sick with TB (Dobler and Marks 2013), but the majority of latent TB infections worldwide do not become active and infectious. Contacts of multidrug-resistant TB patients reportedly have a high risk of developing TB (Fox et al. 2017). Aluni's children fit into that risk category. The switch turning a TB infection into active TB disease, in most cases, is malnutrition. Famine in North Korea between 1994 and 1998, for example, led to a seven-fold increase in TB (Stone 2013). Overcrowded housing, air pollution, and lack of healthcare help spread the disease. But, under healthy conditions, most people with latent TB infection can walk around disease-free unaware of the sleeping microbe inside them. In Daru, where the conditions for TB reactivation are ripe, how long would it be before Aluni's children would fall sick themselves?

In 2020, a staggering 15% of the ten million people worldwide who contracted TB succumbed to the disease. Despite the treatability of TB, the 2022 Global TB report reveals an alarming rise in TB incidence. The underfunding and mismanagement of TB keep the disease at the top of these charts. TB patients and the frontline healthcare staff caring for them are not to be blamed. Significant funding gaps impede efforts to end TB with the Stop TB Partnership and WHO reporting a TB care and Prevention funding gap of $US 2.3 billion in 2017 and a research and development funding gap of $US 1.2 billion per year for the development of new tools. In 2020, only $US 5.3 billion of the necessary $US 13 billion required for TB care and prevention was available and only $US 901 million of the $US 2 billion required for TB research was available (Chakaya et al. 2022). This underfunding maintains the circulation of TB within communities and preserves the high numbers of people with latent TB infections. This situation leads to an unsavoury question: By neglecting latent TB infections, are affluent nations providing sufficient funding for TB health care merely to appear charitable without a genuine commitment to eradicating the disease?

While community-wide screening has helped reduce TB in high-income countries like Australia and The Netherlands (Mason et al. 2016), similar strategies have not been widely implemented in low- and middle-income countries, with a province in Vietnam being one of the few exceptions (Marks et al. 2019). As a result, TB is uncommon in high-income countries but relatively common elsewhere. If a global famine occurs, high-income countries will initially be largely protected, but other countries may become highly susceptible given the existing prevalence of TB.

In 2022, the UN marked the 15th of November as the day human population surpassed eight billion people worldwide. The Malthusian concern regarding overpopulation posits that dwindling resources, if coupled with population growth, will lead to scarcity. This vulnerability is exacerbated in low- and middle-income countries where food insecurity and a high prevalence of TB infection create a precarious situation. The spectre of famine, as evidenced by North Korea's experience, could awaken TB infections, triggering a surge in active cases and potentially causing the global population to plummet. A place like Daru Island would be a tinderbox. When affluent governments neglect treating latent TB infections in low-income settings, is it a case of calculated negligence?

An unnerving possibility emerges: Is latent TB infection being kept as an overpopulation failsafe? Using TB as an overpopulation failsafe is morally unpalatable and positively eugenic. The reluctance to allocate adequate resources for TB eradication prompts a sobering inquiry into whether latent TB infections are considered an inadvertent means of population control. Pointing the finger at world leaders for something they have not done is challenging. By feigning ignorance or misdirecting attention, world leaders could potentially execute this failsafe without directly intervening. The increasing prevalence of TB could then be portrayed as a tragic biological inevitability. Urgent accountability is required; otherwise, leaders might deflect responsibility, claiming innocence in a scenario where the overpopulation failsafe is executed without their explicit involvement. Unless we hold world leaders accountable now, their chilling apathetic refrain might be, "Look, no hands!"

## Acknowledgements

My heartfelt gratitude extends, first, to the individuals who graciously shared their stories, time, and experiences, infusing the research with depth and nuance. The trust placed in us to share this fleeting glimpse into their lives is the cornerstone of this work and I honour their contributions. Special acknowledgement goes to Homiri and Darius, whose dedication went beyond the ordinary to conduct and transcribe semi-structured interviews with current and former TB patients on Daru Island. Their invaluable efforts add layers of authenticity to our understanding. To Camilla Burkot, a maestro of facilitation during fieldwork on Daru Island, your expertise navigated the complexities of the anthropological journey, for which I am immensely grateful. Danielle Corrie, with her meticulous attention to detail, assisted with sorting, compiling, and synthesizing the qualitative data from interviews. Her contribution extends to proofreading the manuscript you hold. Suman Majumdar from the Burnet Institute and Angela Kelly-Hanku from the University of New South Wales, your support in establishing the groundwork for fieldwork and connecting us with key contacts in Papua New Guinea was instrumental. Your collaboration has left an indelible mark on the trajectory of the research. This ethnographic project was made possible by seed funding from the TB-CRE. Ongoing work is funded by the Australian National Health & Medical Research Council (NHMRC) with CIs A.M. Kelly-Hanku, S.M. Graham, A. Vallely, S. Majumdar, B. Marais, W.S. Pomat, and S. Bell. I am grateful for our shared commitment to understanding and addressing the complexities of TB in our global landscape, a project bigger than all of us.

## References

Abubakar, I., Zignol, M., Falzon, D., Raviglione, M., Ditiu, L., Masham, S., Adetifa, I., Ford, N., Cox, H. and Lawn, S.D. (2013) Drug-resistant tuberculosis: time for visionary political leadership. *The Lancet Infectious Diseases*, 13(6), 529–539.

Adepoyibi, T., Keam, T., Kuma, A., Haihuie, T., Hapolo, M., Islam, S., Akumu, B., Chani, K., Morris, L. and Taune, M. (2019) A pilot model of patient education and counselling for drug-resistant tuberculosis in Daru, Papua New Guinea. *Public Health in Action*, 9(Suppl 1), S80–S82. https://doi.org/10.5588/pha.18.0096

Arthur, W.S. (1992) Culture and economy in border regions: the torres strait case. *Australian Aboriginal Studies*, 2, 15–33.

Brimnes, N. (2016) *Languished Hopes: Tuberculosis, the State and International Assistance in Twentieth-century India*. Orient Blackswan, Hyderabad.

Brolan, C.E., Upham, S.J., Hill, P.S., Simpson, G. and Vincent, S.D. (2011) Borderline health: complexities of the Torres Strait treaty. *Medical Journal of Australia*, 195(9), 503–505.

Busilacchi, S., Butler, J.R., Van Putten, I., Maru, Y. and Posu, J. (2018) Asymmetrical development across transboundary regions: the case of the torres strait treaty region (Australia and Papua New Guinea). *Sustainability*, 10(11), 4200.

Cantor, D. (2003) The diseased body. In R. Cooter and J. Pickstone (Eds.), *Companion to Medicine in the Twentieth Century*, Routledge, London, 347–351.

Carel, H., Kidd, I.J. and Pettigrew, R. (2016) Illness as transformative experience. *The Lancet*, 388(10050), 1152–1153.

Chakaya, J., Petersen, E., Nantanda, R., Mungai, B.N., Migliori, G.B., Amanullah, F., ... and Zumla, A. (2022) The WHO global tuberculosis 2021 report–not so good news and turning the tide back to end TB. *International Journal of Infectious Diseases*, 124, S26–S29.

Chaudhry, P. (2020) The politics of distribution. In M. Moran and J. Curth-Bibb (Eds.), *Too Close to Ignore: Australia's Borderland with PNG and Indonesia*, Melbourne University Press, Victoria, pp. 111–141.

Chuengsatiansup, K. and Limsawart, W. (2019) Tuberculosis in the borderlands: migrants, microbes and more-than-human borders. *Palgrave Communications*, 5(1), 1–10.

Degeling, C., Mayes, C., Lipworth, W., Kerridge, I. and Upshur, R. (2015) The political and ethical challenge of multi-drug resistant tuberculosis. *Journal of Bioethical Inquiry*, 12, 107–113.

Dhavan, P., Dias, H.M., Creswell, J. and Weil, D. (2017) An overview of tuberculosis and migration. *The International Journal of Tuberculosis and Lung Disease*, 21(6), 610–623.

Dheda, K. and Migliori, G.B. (2012) The global rise of extensively drug-resistant tuberculosis: is the time to bring back sanatoria now overdue? *The Lancet*, 379(9817), 773–775.

Dobler, C.C. and Marks, G.B. (2013) Risk of tuberculosis among contacts in a low-incidence setting. *European Respiratory Journal*, 41, 1459–1461.

Dobre, A. (2018) Social construction of tuberculosis. *Challenges of the Knowledge Society*, 1032–1037.

Engel, N. (2015) *Tuberculosis in India: A Case of Innovation and Control*. New Delhi, India: Orient Blackswan.

Fairchild, A.L. and Oppenheimer, G.M. (1998) Public health nihilism vs pragmatism: history, politics, and the control of tuberculosis. *American Journal of Public Health*, 88(7), 1105–1117.

Farmer, P. (2003) *Pathologies of Power: Health, Human Rights, and the New War on the Poor*. Berkeley: University of California Press.

Farmer, P. and Kim, J.Y. (1998) Community based approaches to the control of multidrug resistant tuberculosis: introducing "DOTS-plus". *The British Medical Journal*, 317, 671.

Foster, J., Mendez, D., Marais, B.J., Denholm, J.T., Peniyamina, D., and McBryde, E.S. (September 19, 2022) Critical consideration of tuberculosis management of Papua New Guinea nationals and cross-border health issues in the remote torres Strait Islands, Australia. *Tropical Medicine and Infectious Disease*, 7(9), 251. https://doi.org/10.3390/tropicalmed7090251.

Fox, G.J., Anh, N.T., Nhung, N.V., Loi, N.T., Hoa, N.B., Ngoc Anh, L.T., Cuong, N.K., Buu, T.N., Marks, G.B. and Menzies, D. (2017) Latent tuberculous infection in household contacts of multidrug-resistant and newly diagnosed tuberculosis. *The International Journal of Tuberculosis and Lung Disease*, 21(3), 297–302.

Gilpin, C.M., Simpson, G., Vincent, S., O'Brien, T.P., Knight, T.A., Globan, M., Coulter, C. and Konstantinos, A., 2008. Evidence of primary transmission of multidrug-resistant tuberculosis in the Western Province of Papua New Guinea. *Medical Journal of Australia*, 188(3), pp.148–152.

Harper, I. (2010) Extreme condition, extreme measures? Compliance, drug resistance, and the control of tuberculosis. *Anthropology & Medicine*, 17, 201–214.

Hayward, S., Harding, R.M., McShane, H. and Tanner, R. (2018) Factors influencing the higher incidence of tuberculosis among migrants and ethnic minorities in the UK. F1000Research, 7.

Houben, R.M. and Dodd, P.J. (2016) The global burden of latent tuberculosis infection: a re-estimation using mathematical modelling. PLoS Medicine, 13(10), e1002152.

Jops, P., Cowan, J., Kupul, M., Trumb, R.N., Graham, S.M., Bauri, M., Nindil, H., Bell, S., Keam, T., Majumdar, S., Pomat, M.B., Marks, G.B., Kaldor, J., Vallely, A. and Kelly-Hanku, A. (2023) Beyond patient delay, navigating structural health system barriers to timely care and treatment in a high burden TB setting in Papua New Guinea. Global Public Health, 18(1), 2184482.

Jops, P., Kupul, M., Trumb, R.N., Cowan, J., Graham, S.M., Bell, S., Majumdar, S., Nindil, H., Pomat, W., Marais, B., Marks, G., Vallely, A.J., Kaldor, J. and Kelly-Hanku, A. (2022) Exploring tuberculosis riskscapes in a Papua New Guinean 'hotspot'. Qualitative Health Research, 32(11), 1747–1762.

Koch, E. (2013) Free Market Tuberculosis. Nashville, US: Vanderbilt University Press.

Lawrence, D. (1998) Customary exchange in the Torres Strait. Australian Aboriginal Studies, 2, 13–25.

Litvinjenko, S., Magwood, O., Wu, S. and Wei, X. (2023) Burden of tuberculosis among vulnerable populations worldwide: an overview of systematic reviews. The Lancet. Infectious Diseases, 23(12), 1395.

Maciel, E.M.G.D.S., Amancio, J.D.S., Castro, D.B.D. and Braga, J.U. (2018) Social determinants of pulmonary tuberculosis treatment non-adherence in Rio de Janeiro, Brazil. PLoS One, 13(1), e0190578.

Madjid, A., Syafar, M., Arsunan, A.A. and Maria, I.L. (2020) Social determinants and tuberculosis incidents on empowerment case finding in Majene district. Enfermería Clínica, 30, 136–140.

Marks, G.B., Nguyen, N.V., Nguyen, P.T., Nguyen, T.A., Nguyen, H.B., Tran, K.H., ... and Fox, G.J. (2019) Community-wide screening for tuberculosis in a high-prevalence setting. New England Journal of Medicine, 381(14), 1347–1357.

Mason, P.H. (2019) Excluded from reciprocity: tuberculosis, conspicuous consumption and the medicalization of poverty. In Macdonald, H. and Harper (eds), Understanding Tuberculosis and Its Control. London: Routledge, pp. 206–220.

Mason, P.H., Degeling, C. and Denholm, J. (2015) Sociocultural dimensions of tuberculosis: an overview of key concepts. International Journal of Tuberculosis and Lung Disease, 19(10), 1135–1143. https://doi.org/10.5588/ijtld.15.0066

Mason, P.H., Lyttleton, C., Marks, G.B. and Fox, G.J. (2020) The technological imperative in tuberculosis care and prevention in Vietnam. Global Public Health, 15(2), 307–320.

Mason, P.H., Oni, T., Van Herpen, M.M.J.W. and Coussens, A.K. (2016) Tuberculosis prevention must integrate technological and basic care innovation. European Respiratory Journal, 48(5), 1529–1531. https://doi.org/10.1183/13993003.01449-2016

Mason, P.H., Snow, K., Asugeni, R., Massey, P.D. and Viney, K. (2017) Tuberculosis and gender in the Asia-Pacific region. Australian and New Zealand Journal of Public Health, 41(3), 227–229.

McIver, L.J., Kippin, A.N., Parish, S.T. and Whitehead, O.G. (2010) HIV, Malaria and pneumonia in a Torres Strait Islander male — a case report. Communicable Diseases Intelligence, 34, 448–449.

McMillen, C.W. (2015) *Discovering Tuberculosis: A Global History, 1900 to the Present*. New Haven and London: Yale University Press.

Mitchell, E.M., Daftary, A., Craig, G. and Redwood, L. (2018) Measuring TB stigma as part of a syndemic. *TB Stigma*, 282.

Porter, J., Lee, K. and Ogden, J. (2002) The globalisation of DOTS: tuberculosis as a global emergency. In L. Kelley, B. Kent and F. Suzanne (Eds.), *Health Policy in a Globalising World*. Cambridge, UK: Cambridge University Press, pp. 181–194.

Rosenberg, C.E. (1992) Framing disease: illness, society, and history. In C. Rosenberg and J. Golden (Eds.), *Framing Disease: Studies in Cultural History*. New Brunswick: Rutgers University Press xiii–xxvi.

Simandan, D. (2017) Considering neoliberalism, contempt and allostatic load in the social dynamics of tuberculosis. *Journal of Biosocial Science*, 49(4), 557–558.

Simpson, G., Coulter, C., Weston, J., et al. (2011) Drug resistance patterns of MDRTB in the Western Province of Papua New Guinea. *International Journal of Tuberculosis and Lung Disease*, 15, 551–552.

Stone, R. (2013) Public enemy number one. *Science*, 340, 422–425. https://doi.org/10.1126/science.340.6131.422

Teo, A.K.J., Morishita, F., Islam, T., Viney, K., Ong, C.W., Kato, S., Kim, H.J., Liu, Y., Oh, K.H., Yoshiyama, T., Ohkado, A., Rahevar, K., Kawatsu, Y.M., Prem, K., Yi, S., Tran, H.T.G. and Marais, B.J. (2023) Tuberculosis in older adults: challenges and best practices in the Western Pacific Region. *The Lancet Regional Health–Western Pacific*, 36.

Trauer, J.M., Denholm, J.T., Waseem, S., Ragonnet, R. and McBryde, E.S. (2016) Scenario analysis for programmatic tuberculosis control in Western Province, Papua New Guinea. *American Journal of Epidemiology*, 183, 1138–1148.

Zumla, A.I., Gillespie, S.H., Hoelscher, M., Philips, P.P.J., Cole, S.T., Abubakar, I., McHugh, T.D., Schito, M., Maeurer, M. and Nunn, A.J. (2014) New antituberculosis drugs, regimens, and adjunct therapies: needs, advances, and future prospects. *The Lancet Infectious Diseases*, 14(4), pp. 327–340.

Zvonareva, O., van Bergen, W., Kabanets, N., Alliluyev, A. and Filinyuk, O. (2019) Experiencing syndemic: disentangling the biosocial complexity of tuberculosis through qualitative research. *Journal of Biosocial Science*, 51(3), 403–417.

# 4 The rise and fall of India's national tuberculosis programme, 1960–1997

*Niels Brimnes*

## Introduction

It may be useful to think of the history of attempts to control tuberculosis (TB) since the nineteenth century as a series of consecutive but overlapping phases. In the first phase, lasting until World War II, the main intervention was institutional treatment, typically in sanatoria. This type of intervention was expensive and limited to populations in affluent parts of the world and to elites elsewhere. Towards the end of this phase, TB went into a significant decline in Europe and North America, not as a direct result of institutional treatment, but attributable to improving standards of living. A second phase was heralded by the discovery and application of new biomedical remedies – the BCG vaccine and antibiotic drugs – in the first two decades after the war and also character-ized by a shift of the 'tuberculosis problem' towards developing countries. In this phase, TB control was dominated by vertical mass vaccination campaigns and clinically oriented explorations of the potential of the new drugs. The newly established World Health Organization (WHO) emerged as a key agent in these efforts. A third phase began in the early 1960s, when national con-trol programmes incorporating the new remedies were designed throughout the Global South. These programmes were based on simplified versions of biomedical technology and to varying degrees integrated into the general health services. Gradually, the international health establishment, including the WHO, lost interest in TB, which increasingly – and erroneously – came to be seen as a disease of the past. Around 1990 a conjuncture of developments spurred a renewed interest in TB. The worldwide emergence of co-infection with HIV and an unexpected outbreak of multidrug resistant (MDR) TB in New York City combined with economic attention from the World Bank to put TB back on the international health agenda and caused a major and rather sudden reorientation of the efforts to control the disease. In this fourth phase, global TB control became synonymous with the so-called DOTS programme, which was technically based on significantly shorter drug regimens and organizationally based on upgraded infrastructure and intensified supervision. At the turn of the twenty-first century, TB control became, therefore, more

DOI: 10.4324/9781032634647-4

narrowly bio-medical, standardized, vertical, and even paternalistic, but also significantly better funded.[1]

Within this frame, the development of the Indian National Tuberculosis Programme (NTP) stands out as emblematic for the third phase. In the 1960s, the Indian programme was highlighted as an inspirational model for developing countries across the world, while 30 years later, the transition into the DOTS phase of TB control was both controversial and disputed. This chapter narrates the trajectory of this pivotal programme.[2] By delving into the history of the Indian NTP, this chapter highlights the interconnectedness of global TB control efforts and the ways in which experiences in one country can inform policies and practices globally. As TB remains a significant global health challenge, understanding the nuances of TB control programmes in diverse settings is essential for shaping effective and equitable strategies at the international level.

Overall, the inclusion of a chapter on the Indian NTP enriches the narrative of the global history of TB by providing a nuanced examination of TB control efforts in a key country, offering valuable insights into the evolution of TB control strategies and their impact on broader public health initiatives worldwide.

## A new departure in TB control

While it is difficult to determine exactly when the Indian National Tuberculosis programme began, the inauguration of the National Tuberculosis Institute (NTI) in Bangalore (now Bengaluru) in September 1960 is an obvious starting point. The atmosphere was enthusiastic on this festive occasion, attended by several dignitaries including Jawaharlal Nehru, and there was a sense that something new was beginning. P. V. Benjamin, the respected doyen of TB control in India, confidently declared that the new institute was "a departure from orthodox procedures" and that "a totally new idea is going to take shape" (National Tuberculosis Institute 2000).[3]

While it was clear that this new departure in TB control was going to be very different from the unrealistic focus on providing institutional treatment, which had prevailed before the war, the relationship with the bio-medical breakthroughs in recent decades was more ambiguous. The new approach should obviously build on the perceived success of the mass BCG vaccination campaign in India – perhaps the largest vaccination effort in history – which had been conducted throughout the 1950s. But mass vaccination was set to terminate in 1961, and it was understood that future vaccination efforts ought to be integrated either into a broader TB control framework or into the general health services. The general view was that the days of the top-down vertical intervention were gone, and a more horizontal approach had to take over (Brimnes 2016).[4]

Similarly, the time had come to take the new wonder-drugs out of the clinical set-up, in which they had been tested and their potential determined. In this clinical effort, the Tuberculosis Chemotherapy Centre in Madras (now Chennai) had been crucial. Established in 1956 with Wallace Fox from the British Medical Research Council as Director, the centre had shown that regimens of new antibiotic drugs were as efficient when taken in the homes of poor tubercular patients as when taken in hospitals and sanatoria. These important results were published in 1959 and promised to turn TB into a curable disease, also – notably – for poor people in developing countries (Bulletin of WHO 1959).[5] From a curative point of view at least, TB might be able to shed its dreaded label as a 'social disease'. Another publication from the Madras Centre phrased it in this way: "the successful treatment of patients in their homes need not await an increase in the standard of living" (Ramakrishnan et al. 1961).[6]

It was, however, one thing to demonstrate the theoretical feasibility of domiciliary chemotherapy in a clinical trial, conducted in the convenient vicinity of a research centre; it was quite another to design a programme that would make this type of treatment work under field conditions throughout India and even beyond. To meet this challenge was the *raison d'etre* behind the establishment of NTI: its most important task was to transform the results from the vertical vaccination campaigns and clinical drug trials of the 1950s into a programme suited to the field conditions in India. According to one of the main architects of the programme, the doctor and sociologist Debabar Banerji, the programme should be: "nationally applicable, socially acceptable, and epidemiologically effective" (Banerji 2017).[7] This transformative task was not lost on Benjamin. In a 1961 account of the attempt to control TB in India, he (1961) wrote:

> Till recently, the generally accepted methods of tuberculosis control were mainly confined to a clinical approach in which the clinician had the most important part to play, his chief concern being the individual patient, his diagnosis and treatment ... The new approach now being worked out is meant to tackle the problem on a community basis where the preventive and social aspects will have a prominent place.[8]

With this quote, Benjamin explicitly distanced himself from individualized – and costly – clinical treatment in institutions, but he also suggested that the clinical trials of domiciliary treatment had done their job. It was time to move in a new, community-oriented direction.

## Designing the programme

In the years following the inauguration of NTI, several important decisions were taken, based on epidemiological and – perhaps surprisingly – also sociological research carried out by NTI. A rare sight in public health institutions in the developing world around 1960, the NTI had a significant sociological section, headed by Banerji, who was trained as a medical doctor, but employed as a sociologist by NTI in late 1959. Banerji praised the intellectual environment at NTI in the early years as stimulating and genuinely cross-disciplinary. In his autobiography, he also refers to the "deep friendship" he developed with two Danish WHO officers: Stig Andersen, his international sociologist counterpart, and Halfdan Mahler, the Senior Medical Officer (Banerji 2017; Brimnes 2023).[9] Mahler would later become a significant Director General of the WHO between 1973 and 1988 and particularly remembered for his strong commitment to the 'Primary Health Care' strategy, which incorporated ideas similar to those which were developed at NTI. Around 1960 Bangalore was indeed a special and innovative place in global TB control.

An early and important decision was that the NTP would be based on passive case-finding through sputum microscopy. The preference for passive case-finding was based on the view that a sufficiently large number of patients would report to the health services on their own initiative, and that there was no reason to spend additional resources on actively identifying more patients than the system had the capacity to treat. According to Andersen, the basic philosophy of the programme was, that "it is the first obligation of a tuberculosis programme to take care of those cases which are now standing at the very door-step of the health services, seeking assistance". This was also frequently referred to as the 'felt need' approach. Sputum microscopy was preferred to X-ray diagnostic because it was cheaper, simpler, and only identified infectious, sputum-positive patients. While it could be argued that diagnosis through X-ray would identify more patients in an earlier stage of disease, and therefore enhance the probability of successful treatment, the counter-argument was that it risked clogging the system with un- or less infective patients, and even – as X-ray diagnosis was less precise than microscopy – with patients not suffering from TB (Anderson 1963).[10]

Another decision determined the drug regimen, which should be administered to the patients. The premise was that the drugs provided through the NTP had to be free of costs, and the clinical trials from Madras suggested a combination therapy of the cheapest and easiest available anti-TB drug, Isoniazid (INH), with the much more expensive PAS. Despite strong desires to base a TB control programme on treatment with INH alone, PAS was added to both enhance efficacy and curb the emergence of resistant bacteria. These advantages came, however, with prohibitive costs. When the official recommendations for a district TB programme were circulated in 1962, they declared that "it should be the definite policy to treat all cases who are infectious, that is, sputum positive, with two drugs", but immediately added: "In the absence of two drugs Isoniazid alone may be given". Accepting the financial realities in India in the 1960s, WHO Medical Officer Maurice Piot explained how the entire budget for anti-TB drugs in the third five-year plan (covering the period 1961–1966) had to be spent on the cheap INH, and added that "the cost of a programme based on combined therapy, however, desirable, remains today prohibitive ...". Being well-aware of the scientific reason to insist on multi-drug therapy, the designers India's NTP pragmatically decided that 'one is better than none' (Piot 1962).[11]

A third decision was that the NTP had to be based on patient's self-administration of drugs. Effective treatment required that patients took the prescribed drugs regularly over 12 months, even though they would start feeling much better after a few weeks of treatment. Moreover, it was important that patient did not stop treatment prematurely, because this would accelerate the development of drug resistance. This was the classic 'defaulter' problem and a major challenge, formulated by a WHO study group in 1957 through two pertinent questions:

> To what extent will uneducated an entirely asymptomatic patients continue to take any single or multiple drug regimen, irrespective of palatability, and for how long? Will the efforts necessary to ensure a reasonable degree of such long-continued co-operation prove to be administratively feasible?
> (WHO 1957)[12]

This classic dilemma invited extended discussions about the need for some degree of supervision to secure patient compliance. The clinical trials conducted by the Madras Centre boasted impressive results in this area, but this was due to plentiful resources and not replicable under field conditions. Eventually, and once again guided by pragmatic acceptance of financial and infrastructural limitations, the designers of NTP opted for non-supervised, self-administration of drugs. Patients were expected to collect their drugs once a month on their own initiative and stay on a treatment that prescribed a daily intake of unpleasant drugs for a year. If a patient did not turn up to collect medicine a home visit would be paid, and after two unsuccessful home visits, the patient would be considered a 'final defaulter' (Anderson and Banerji 1963).[13]

In the discussion about patient regularity, the sociologists at the NTI played an important role in shifting the blame from the 'ignorant and superstitious' patient to the public health infrastructure. As mentioned above, Fox and his team had maintained a high level of compliance in the Madras trials, because they had been able to commit resources to supervision and tracing. Fox obviously knew that this model was not feasible in a nationwide programme. He also understood the constraints that prevented desperately poor patients from skipping work and travelling significant distances to obtain their drugs, but he remained focussed on the shortcomings of the individual patient. In 1958 – after comparing the typical patient with the average individual who easily "forgets or fails to clean his teeth" – he speculated: "In essence, in order to make a patient take medicine regularly morning and night for a year it is necessary to establish a new pattern of behaviour; and this many of our patients find difficult" (Fox 1958).[14] It was this focus and its ensuing pessimism that Andersen and Banerji challenged in an article in the *Bulletin of the WHO* in 1963. According to the two NTI sociologists, the key problem in securing patient regularity lay not with the defaulting individual, but in programme infrastructure:

> The essential finding of the present study is that the straightforward defaulter problem, the classical problem of discontinuation of chemotherapy, is actually a *smaller* problem than the combination of a number of other administrative and organizational problems, as shown above.

Somewhat more optimistically than Fox, they concluded that organizational and administrative improvements could deal with "a considerable proportion of losses of patents" and that straightforward defaulting could be "very considerably reduced" by the same measures (Anderson and Banerji 1963).[15]

A final decision to be taken concerned the future of BCG vaccination, but this turned out to be a decision never taken. Despite a rhetorical commitment to integrate BCG into a broader frame, such integration was repeatedly deemed premature, and the actual type of integration was uncertain. No admirer of the vertical campaign, even Mahler – who began his career in WHO as supervisor of mass BCG vaccination – expressed reluctance. In 1955, in his last report as supervisor to the Indian mass BCG campaign, he described integration as "at best a wistful truism" and declared that the present vertical set-up had to continue "till such time which we have achieved a satisfactory epidemiological coverage". Five years later, the NTI oscillated between recommending integration and accepting continued mass vaccination. In 1961, a report argued that the mass campaign had "lost its initial momentum", and that some of the arguments for a specialized vaccination effort "no longer had same compelling urgency" as when the mass vaccination was initiated in a decade earlier. Yet, one year later, however, NTI accepted that it was still premature to attempt to integrate BCG (Mahler 1955).[16]

As these fundamental questions about the proper design of TB control programme were being settled, the Union Government approved a set of recommendations for district TB programmes, envisaged to be the basic operational unit of the effort to control the disease. This, it could be argued, was the real beginning of the NTP.[17] Also in 1962, WHO Medical Officer Maurice Piot laid out the basic principles behind the programme in *The Indian Journal of Tuberculosis*. Piot declared that a reasonable target of the programme was a 50% reduction of the number of infectious, sputum-positive cases in 20 years, and emphasized that the programme was the result of an attempt "… to strike a balance between what is technically desirable and what is operationally (including financially) feasible". The NTP was, in other words, a programme full of compromises. Piot (1962) also highlighted the integrated and community-oriented nature of the NTP:

> The important elements of the plan are thought to be (a) the highest possible degree of integration of the tuberculosis programme into the general

public health services (especially the Primary Health Units) and (b) the maximum participation of the local Government (Panchayats) and of the Community Development Department.

Stig Andersen (1961) reached a similar conclusion in one of his reports to the WHO. Through its endorsement of the District Tuberculosis Programmes (DTP), the Indian authorities had:

> ... formally adopted the policy that the prevention and treatment of tuberculosis is the task of all general public health services and that tuberculosis control in India shall be developed, not as a specialised service dedicated to a fortunate few who live near TB clinics, but in consonance with, indeed as part of, the expansion and improvement of the basic rural and urban health services.

## Running the programme

The programme that was rolled out from 1962 was envisaged as a three-tier structure. At the apex, the NTI conducted research and trained key personnel to man the programme throughout India. At the level of the Indian states, Tuberculosis Control Centres relieved the NTI of the more basic training activities and supervised the programme at the district level. In each district, a TB centre would be responsible for running the Tuberculosis District Programme (DTP). A district centre had a staff of 13, including a BCG vaccination team, laboratory facilities for sputum microscopy and an X-ray unit. Even if the vaccination team was formally attached to the centre, its mode of operation was still the vertical mass campaign. (Piot 1961) Below the district centre, the NTP was entirely integrated into the general public health infrastructure, and it was expected that most cases would be diagnosed by multipurpose health workers in sub-district 'Public Health Units' (later renamed 'Peripheral Health Institutions'). This was seen as a realistic programme suited to the conditions prevailing on the ground in India – and in other developing countries throughout the world.

Therefore, when WHO's expert committee on TB – with Mahler serving as its secretary – issued its eighth report in 1964, the Indian programme was easily recognizable in the text. First, the report emphasized that developing countries should not imitate the control strategies employed in "technically advanced" countries. The Committee recommended, instead, "that all financial resources and manpower available for tuberculosis control in the developing countries be confined to organizing efficient ambulatory services and not to construct new beds". It further recommended to continue BCG vaccination on a mass scale in countries where TB was a serious problem. These recommendations were in line with the general framework of the Indian programme, and the report also referred to its more specific features. Mentioning sociological enquiries into the awareness of symptoms among patients, which suggested that such an awareness had been underestimated, was an obvious reference to Banerji's and Andersen's research. It employed the concept of 'felt need', and it accepted that circumstances might exist, in which the only feasible option was to provide mono-drug treatment with INH. When the committee concluded that "an effective national tuberculosis programme is possible under any given situation, provided application is guided by sound principles …", few were in doubt that this optimism was based on the efforts carried out at the NTI and operationalized in the NTP. By the mid-1960s, the Indian programme seemed destined to conquer the world (WHO 1964).[18]

On the ground, however, things did not develop as smoothly as hoped. A first challenge was to extend the programme throughout the country. The ambition was to have a recognized programme in all of India's districts by the end of the fourth five-year plan in 1971. Until 1966, the programme did expand at an increasing pace, but not fast enough. By 1965, WHO Medical officer D. Savic found "quite a mountain to climb", as 85 districts had a recognized programme running according to the official guidelines. In 1966, a record 42 new district programmes were added, but then the expansion slowed down, and by the 1980s a fifth of India's 400 districts were still without a programme. Below the district centres coverage was lower. In 1969, for instance, only half of the Peripheral Health Institutions offered the TB services, which were supposed to be an integrated part of the general health services (Brimnes 2016).[19] The Indian states, that enjoyed extensive autonomy in the district levels, turned out to be reluctant collaborator, and the establishment of State Tuberculosis Control Centres was unsatisfactory. This created, according to one observer a 'vacuum' between district services and central institutions and meant that the NTP was not properly supervised. The lack of systematic evaluation of the programme was defined as a major failure of the programme by Andersen early as 1963 and would later be a point of severe criticism (Brimnes 2016).[20]

The NTP also struggled to identify a satisfactory number of patients. From the late 1960s, it was decided that the 'satisfactory' performance of an average DTP was to diagnose 400 patients each quarter, but most DTPs struggled to meet that target. Figures from the late 1970s show that it was common for a DTP to diagnose less than 100 patients per quarter. In 1981, the general performance of the programme, measured against the target of 400 diagnosed patients per quarter, was below 40%. Unsurprisingly, the main problem was the Peripheral Health Institutions beyond the district headquarters. This meant that – contrary to the intentions behind the programme – the NTP worked much better in urban than in rural areas.

The supply of free drugs created problems from the inception of the programme and remained erratic throughout its lifetime. As early as in 1962, there was a shortage of PAS, and in 1964 the Government of India was so concerned about the drug supply, that it converted its financial commitment towards the running of the NTP infrastructure into the procurement of drugs. As domestic drug production was insufficient, UNICEF assisted with drugs produced abroad and in 1965 further agreed to supply virtually the entire programme with the cheap and basic isoniazid for two years. In 1968, it was estimated that the stock of PAS was sufficient for a third of the patients that were supposed to take it, and in 1969 UNICEF again had to intervene to avoid an acute shortage of isoniazid. Unsurprisingly, the TB advisor to the Government of India and former director of NTI, N. L. Bordia, in 1967 referred to drug supply as the "weak link in the chain of measures" that should keep the NTP going. Despite the arrival of new drugs such as in the 1970s and 1980s, supply problems seem to have persisted. Continuous problems with the supply of drugs meant, therefore, that monotherapy with isoniazid must have continued to be widespread in the NTP (Bordia 1967).[21]

Finally, patient compliance remained unsatisfactory in the NTP. Whether it was due to patient behaviour or infrastructural weaknesses, too few patients completed their 12-month self-administered treatment. Even at NTIs 'model' site in Anantapur in Andhra Pradesh – used for educational purposes – the rate of defaulters was in some areas up to 50% in the early 1960s. Twenty years later the recorded general rate of compliance in the programme was just below 30% (NTP 1988).[22] The low compliance rate was not just making the programme less successful in alleviating the TB problem in India, it also combined with erratic drug supply to enhance the emergence of resistance and thus create new problems in the effort to control TB. The resistance problem had been known since the discovery of antibiotics and was regularly reported among TB patients in India. Studies conducted both by NTI and the Indian Council of Medical Research suggested that up 20% of patients carried bacteria resistant to isoniazid. A significant part of this was pre-treatment (or primary) resistance, which indicated that resistant strains of bacteria circulated among the Indian population. The experts – whether Indian or international – did not, seem particularly worried. A 1973 study from New Delhi found pre-treatment resistance in 17.5% of the patients but concluded that it was not an important factor in treatment failure. This view echoed the opinion voiced by Wallace Fox the year before in an article based on results from a BMRC trial in Hong Kong. There were, however, some rare warnings. One came from WHO-consultant Karel Styblo, who would later play a crucial role in the development of the DOTS programme. In 1971, Styblo together with his colleague Stefan Grzybowsky concluded that treatment regimens based on isoniazid and streptomycin or – even worse – isoniazid alone aggravated the development of drug-resistance. They advised that they be substituted by available regimens based on other drugs but such a change took many years to come.[23]

## Reviewing the programme

As the NTP struggled to live up expectation, several critical reviews were conducted. An ICMR review from 1975 noted that its performance had been far from satisfactory and recommended among other things the posting of more specialized TB staff below the district centres (Brimnes 2016).[24] A decade later the Bangalore-based NGO, ICORCI, was commissioned to conduct an 'in depth study' of the programme. ICORCI submitted an extensive report in 1988 which pointed out that the programme was underperforming on several parameters: case detection was too low to have a significant impact on India's TB problem, treatment completion rates were unsatisfactory, and not enough attention was given to defaulting patients. The picture was, therefore, "quite gloomy" (ICORCI 1988).[25] The report drew particular attention to the fact that X-ray diagnosis seemed to be preferred over the simpler and more reliable sputum microscopy. This was a significant deviation, not only from the original NTP guideline, but also from the official WHO recommendation. Preference for X-ray led to significant over-treatment, which was both uneconomical and unethical and described as a "crime against society".[26] The report also criticized supervision within and monitoring of the programme. Adequate supervision of activities below the district centre was "almost non-existing", while programme officers expressed the feeling that NTP had become a neglected programme, receiving both less funding and less attention from the authorities compared to other programmes.[27]

Despite these shortcomings the ICORCI study was fundamentally loyal to the foundational principles of the NTP. This was in accordance with the assignment given to the NGO, which was to review the programme "in accordance with its basic principles", not to question these principles.[28] This loyalty became clear in the report's treatment of the integration of the NTP into the general health services. This was an obviously problematic element in the programme. The report noted how tasks related to TB did not become part of the job description for local health workers in the general health services until the 1980s, how these workers had insufficient knowledge of TB symptoms, how half of them did not participate in case finding activities, and how instruction in manuals from the general health services diverged from the manuals issued by NTI. The report also regretted that multi-purpose health workers had recently been deprived of the task of conducting sputum tests (ICORCI 1988).[29]

Despite this long list of issues, ICORCI did not turn against the principle of integration. The report saw the problems as indications "of the travails of integration", supported the ambition of the bringing hitherto disconnected personnel engaged in "unipurpose activities" together in an integrated system, and found it "not surprising that the process of integration is still not fully completed at all levels".[30] While the level case finding at local health institutions was desperately low, it was actually improving, and the report saw this as "a very healthy trend in decentralisation of diagnostic facilities". In a similar vein, the report recommended that the task of collecting sputum samples were given back to local multipurpose workers, as this was "the only way of meeting the sociological objective of providing services close to the homes of the people".[31] In this way, the 1988 review remained faithful to the values of both integration and decentralization of TB services, which had guided the establishment of the NTP 25 years earlier.

It would be only a few years until another – shorter and sharper – review was conducted in 1992; this time by the WHO, the Government of India, and the Swedish development aid agency (SIDA). The 1992 review identified many of the same flaws in the programme. It found an over-reliance on X-ray diagnosis, whereas the proportion of bacteriologically confirmed cases was "extremely low", and it described recording and monitoring within the programme as "seriously deficient". In line with the ICORCI report, the 1992 review found that the NTP had considerable basic strengths, but also that the original philosophy of decentralization and integration had neither been fully implemented nor appropriately revised over three decades (TPR 1992).[32]

The 1992 review also drew attention to new issues. It criticized that the NTP had functioned without monitoring the rates of treatment completion and cure, and recommended that registration practices be revised to enable this kind of surveillance. Among the nine major recommendations highlighted in the review was that the hitherto neglected cure rate ought to serve as "the main indicator of programme effectiveness" (TPR 1992).[33] The review also recommended the introduction of new and more sophisticated regimens of short course therapy (SCCs), which would bring the duration of treatment down to six–eight months. While the ICORCI review had noted how SCCs were being introduced in some places and urged the NTP to make a general decision on whether to use them or not; the 1992 review was unambiguously in favour of introducing them as speedily as possible (ICORCI 1988).[34]

The review also addressed two emerging issues that would define the global TB control agenda in decades to come: co-infection with HIV and drug resistance. The review recognized that co-infection with HIV was a future concern, but had found no evidence that it impacted the current situation. It was, therefore, confident that co-infected HIV-TB patients would "represent only a fraction" of TB patients in the coming decade.[35] The review was more concerned about drug resistance. It found the level of secondary (acquired) resistance to both rifampicin and isoniazid "particularly serious".[36]

This all added up to a general verdict, which was similar to the one given by ICORCI four years earlier, but now expressed in stronger terms. The programme was seen as "not having a measurable impact" on the transmission of TB in India and "to function far below its potential". The review found "no evidence of a significant decrease in TB during the last three decades" and looked into a future that was significantly 'gloomier' than the one presented by ICORCI's (1988) four years earlier:

> An aging population structure, increasing HIV prevalence and apparently rising levels of drug resistance mean that without a reoriented and vitalized public TB control effort the disease will pose an increasingly serious health and developmental constraint for several decades to come ....

At the same time, however, the 1992 review represented not only a re-discovery of TB as a serious public health problem, but also as a field that merited significant investment. Perhaps the most important criticism forwarded by the review was that the TB programme had languished at the national level in the Ministry of Health, where it ranged below other programmes and where several key positions were vacant. One consequence was that programme management had been ceded to the NTI, although the institute neither had the staff nor the executive authority to assume this role. The first (1992) of the major recommendations were, therefore:

> 1) establishing an apex policy making authority and an executive task force with managerial functions to implement programme reorganization and 2) upgrading the central tuberculosis control unit in the Directorate [General of Health Services] to provide strong leadership and enhance the efficiency and effectiveness of the National Tuberculosis Programme.

This was combined with a recognition that – after decades of relative neglect – it was worthwhile to invest in TB control. Given that the burden from TB mortality in India was described as both staggering and enormous, the review emphasized that "the discounted cost per healthy year of life gained as a result of a well-functioning tuberculosis control programme will be well under US $10, making tuberculosis control one of the highest priority interventions for the State and central government" (TRP 1992). The last sentence of the review clearly conveyed the notion that TB control had become a good investment, also for foreign donors: "Given the demonstrated cost-effectiveness of TB control programmes compared to other health sector interventions, revision and expansion of India's TB programme with external financial assistance would appear to be fully justified". It seemed that TB control in India had moved from being based on the 'felt need' in the population to being justified through cost-efficiency.

Finally, the 1992 review suggested that TB control in India had stagnated, and that it would be appropriate to send Indian TB workers abroad. This would, the review claimed, "accelerate adoption of effective new experience in TB control elsewhere".[37] It also seemed, therefore, that India, which for decades had provided the model programme for other developing countries, was now going to import approaches developed in other regions.

## Challenging the programme

The profound challenges to India's approach to TB control around 1990 must indeed be understood in relation to a conjuncture of developments taking place elsewhere: most importantly in East Africa and World Bank Headquarters. In the late 1970s – when TB control was seriously out of fashion in international health – the International Union Against Tuberculosis and

Lung Disease (IUALTD) became involved in the development of a national TB programme in Tanzania. A key figure in this endeavour was the Union's Director of Research, Karel Styblo, who had visited India as a WHO consultant in 1971 and warned against the risk of developing drug resistance as a result of inadequate drug regimens. In Tanzania, however, Styblo oversaw a programme that initially prioritized operational improvements over medical sophistication. The main focus was on better reporting within the programme and systematic registration of patients and treatment outcome. As the historian Christoph Gradmann (2019; 2020) has noted, the Tanzanian programme appeared in its early days as "an interesting mix of organizational innovation and pharmaceutical traditionalism".[38] The programme was launched as integrated with the general health services, but it soon developed several features of a specialized, vertical health intervention. Almost immediately the programme adopted observed treatment, and from 1982 it introduced the more sophisticated short-course regimens (SCCs). With the adoption of these regimens came hospitalization in the first two months, when patients were most infective. By dismissing BCG vaccination as an effective tool in TB control, the Tanzanian programme also prioritized cure over prevention.[39]

All these features ran counter, not only to the principles underpinning the Indian NTP but also to the general WHO policy, which evolved around the concept of primary health care and prioritized simple technologies and integrated programmes. In 1982–1983, it came to a direct conflict between the Union and the WHO. The Union sent a letter to WHO Director-General Mahler criticizing the established policy on TB control. Mahler, of course, was a major stakeholder in the existing approach: he had been one of the architects of the Indian programme, which informed the current WHO policy and conformed to the director-General's signature project: the vision of primary health care. Unsurprisingly, Mahler and WHO dismissed the approach developed in Tanzania as being incompatible with this vision (Gradman 2019).

In 1993 the World Bank published its landmark report 'Investing in Health', which marked the Bank's entrance as a major player in global health. Soaked in rhetoric about cost-efficiency, the report introduced the concept of 'Disability Adjusted Life-Years' (DALY). This was an attempt to measure the impact of a specific health intervention in the long term and in relation to the national economy. According to the report (1993), good health was "a crucial part of well-being, but spending on health can also be justified on purely economic grounds".[40] It is obvious to see to the calculations made in relation to the Tanzanian programme as a precursor to the concept of DALY, but passages in the 1992 review of the Indian NTP also bore a close resemblance to the way DALY was represented in the World Bank report. Based on calculations on cost-efficiency, chemotherapy against TB was repeatedly mentioned as a highly cost-efficient intervention, which should be part of a package of 'essential clinical services' envisaged to be the backbone of public health in developing countries (World Bank 1993).[41]

At this point, the WHO was also shifting its position. Mahler had stepped down as Director-General in 1988 and the commitment to the primary health-care strategy faded after his departure.[42] The new head of the WHOs TB section, Arata Kochi, was sympathetic towards the approach developed by the Union in Tanzania. In 1991, he presented a new WHO TB control strategy, which referred explicitly to "excellent results" in the form of cure rates above 80% obtained in four countries – including Tanzania – with technical and financial support of the Union. Key elements in the new WHO strategy were to obtain a cure rate of 85% in developing countries, through the adoption of the short-course regimens and rigorous monitoring of treatment results (Kochi 1991).[43]

Probably fuelled by the emergence of more and more resistant cases in places like New York City, the TB completed a remarkable come-back in global health. In 1993, as the World Bank highlighted the cost-efficiency of short-course chemotherapy, the WHO declared TB to be global emergency. The following year it published the report 'TB – A Global Emergency', noting that TB was the world's most deadly infectious disease, quoting the World Bank's report to the effect that "TB control" was among the most cost-effective health interventions available, and highlighting Tanzania's model programme. According to the report (WHO 1994) "Tanzania's success can be credited to its adherence to the treatment guidelines now recommended by WHO and pioneered by the International Union Against TB and Lung Disease".[44] Within a decade the WHO had made a complete U-turn in relation to the TB control strategy developed by the Union in Tanzania. What had been dismissed in 1983 was now unreservedly embraced. India, by contrast, hardly figured in the report.

While the acronym DOTS ('Directly Observed Treatment Short-course') was not employed in 'TB – A Global emergency', the report essentially contained the five elements normally associated with the strategy: (1) sustained government commitment to TB control, (2) case detection through sputum microscopy of self-reporting patients, (3) standardized and directly observed short course treatment, (4) regular supply of essential drugs, and (5) a reporting system that allowed systematic assessment of treatment result.[45] The DOTS 'package' came to India in 1993 when pilot programmes were implemented, and in 1997 – after the Government of India had obtained significant funding from the World Bank – the Revised National Tuberculosis Programme (RNTCP) was launched.[46] The days of the once celebrated Indian NTP were over.

## Standing up for the national TB programme

If it seemed that public health experts across the world unanimously rallied behind the new approach to TB control, this was not the case in India. Debabar Banerji – one of the architects behind the NTP and professor at the Centre for Social medicine and Community Health at Jawaharlal Nehru University – protested loudly. In 1992, he delivered an oration for India's TB workers on the 'social science approach' employed to control TB in India. He situated the NTP within an "endogenous body of knowledge" and proudly referred to the "rich heritage of tuberculosis work in India". He commended the programme for putting people before technology, for focussing on the 'felt need' in the population and for 'demystifying' medical knowledge. The NTP represented a proportionate and affordable intervention, it was integrated with general health services, and it would therefore "sink or sail" with their development. It not only conformed to the ideals of primary health care as expressed in the Alma-Ata declaration; Mahler had in 1985 declared that "the health philosophy generated at the NTI had led straight into the concepts used in the Alma-Ata Declaration". By any reckoning, Banerji (1993) concluded, India's contribution to TB control could be considered "an outstanding chapter in the history of public health".[47]

There was no denying, however, that all was not well with the NTP. Banerji provided a narrative of decline from the "idealism and commitment" in the first decades after independence. Specialized, vertical programmes caused a "hemorrhage of resources" from less favoured programmes such as the NTP, and from the mid-1960s political leadership began to "abdicate its responsibilities" in health. These developments damaged the general health services – with which the programme was supposed to 'sink or sail' – and caused "very serious problems in the implementation of the NTP". According to Banerji (1993), the breakdown of India's public health system led to a "collective amnesia" of India's proud heritage in TB work, and to an unfortunate receptiveness to technocentric solutions such as the introduction of the expensive drug rifampicin and short course chemotherapy. And further threats were gathering on the horizon, including the new approach to TB developed by "WHO, World Bank, and some affluent countries". He noted that the WHO and the World Bank had recently invested significantly in TB control in China but insisted that India should reject similar offers.

Banerji's oration was delivered while the NTP was still under assessment, the World Bank had not yet published its landmark report, and the WHO not yet declared TB a global emergency. Four years later, in 1996, Banerji's worst fears had been confirmed. India was on the brink of launching a DOTS-based revised TB control strategy in line with WHO and World Bank recommendations. This caused two concerned NGOs, to commission the now retired Banerji to write an extensive position paper.

This paper reiterated many of the points made in the 1992 oration, but it was also influenced by the new context. The NTP was again described as a laudable result of the "'golden decades' of health service developments in India", and it was duly noted how the WHO had adopted the Indian programme as paradigmatic in 1964. Due to the 'sickness' of the general public health services, however, the NTP has also fallen sick, and it was now in a "very disturbing state" (Banerji 1997).[48] To this narrative of decline, Banerji now added a narrative of betrayal. He accused the affluent countries of having made "a coordinated effort with the WHO and the World Bank to 'forget' the NTP and to impose in its place the RNTCP on India". The hidden agenda of the North was to inflict irrational and costly control measures on the rest of the world, because they were "deadly scared" by the unexpected return of TB to their own countries. The new strategy was 'oblivious' to the valuable research base stemming from India, and instead modelled over Styblo's work in East Africa and the American experience from New York City. This was clearly also a question of self-esteem. To import foreign models was a hard for Indians proud of their own heritage: "To those who had been involved in the NTP since its very inception", the 'foreign' programme came, therefore, not just as an anticlimax, but also as "a form of national humiliation".[49]

Looking beyond issues of betrayal and pride, it is striking that Banerji consistently challenged the cost-efficiency of the RNTCP with references to a natural decline in the incidence of TB. If the epidemiological curve of TB was already declining, it would be ill-advised to force India into a costly programme that would only marginally sharpen this decline. In accordance with this assumption, Banerji declared that the NTP was "conceptualized principally to alleviate suffering caused to the people due to pulmonary TB, it was not visualised as a control programme – a programme meant to reduce the pool of infectors and infection".[50] Banerji noted that the total number of AIDS patients in India was lower than the daily number dying of TB and saw co-infection as yet another problem of the global North imposed on the global health agenda. Similarly, Banerji claimed that the levels of drug resistance in India were insignificant. With reference to the Canadian epidemiologist – and former WHO consultant – Stefan Grzybowski, he claimed that fear of resistance from mono-therapy or poor treatment was "at least exaggerated" (Banerji 1997).[51] While these assumptions were controversial, they firmly place Banerji's perspective on TB in the third phase of TB control, as outlined in the introduction. That it before the fear of co-infection and rising levels of drug resistance entered and altered the equation (Banerji 1997).[52]

## Concluding remarks

It is beyond the scope of this chapter – and beyond the competence of this author – to judge the medical and epidemiological benefits of and problems with both the NTP and the DOTS-based strategies. The latter approach certainly has its own problems and has been criticized in several ways: as a vertical technological fix, as paternalistic, as exacerbating drug resistance, and as the medicalization of poverty (Engel 2014).[53] It might be noted, however, that some of the principles established in Bangalore in the early 1960s continued into the DOTS-based programmes 30 years later: passive case-finding, the use of sputum microscopy to identify infective cases, and the importance of a regular supply of free drugs. From a historian's point of view, the NTP is a hugely important health intervention; but the importance is not only determined by the extent to which it succeeded in reducing the burden of TB in India or beyond. It is also important because it was emblematic of a phase in TB control, when it was assumed that the disease would recede with development and improved standards of life. Rational control programmes were, therefore, integrated with the general health services and could be pragmatic and full of compromises. It belonged to a world before the threats of AIDS and multi-drug resistance made this approach infeasible.

## Notes

1 C. Beaudevin, J. P. Gaudillière, C. Gradmann, A.M. Lowell and L. Pordie, 2020, Global health and the new world order: Introduction, in J. P. Gaudillière, C. Beaudevin, C. Gradmann, A.M. Lowell and L. Pordie (eds.) Global Health and the New World Order. Manchester: Manchester University Press, pp. 1–28; Raviglione, M.C. and Pio, A., 2002. Evolution of WHO policies for tuberculosis control, 1948–2001. *The Lancet, 359*(9308), pp. 775–780; Ogden, J., Walt, G. and Lush, L., 2003. The politics of 'branding'in policy transfer: the case of DOTS for tuberculosis control. Social science & medicine, 57(1), pp. 179–188; Engel, N., 2020. Standardization and localization in tuberculosis control. In Global health and the new world order, in J.P. Gaudillière, C. Beaudevin, C. Gradmann, A.M. Lowell and L. Pordie, (eds), Global Health and the New World Order, Manchester: Manchester University Press. pp. 29–51.

2 The subsequent three sections build substantially on Chapters 6 and 7 in my *Languished Hopes. Tuberculosis, the State and International Assistance in Twentieth Century India* (New Delhi: Orient BlackSwan, 2016).

3 Quoted in *Annals of the National Tuberculosis Institute, Bangalore: 40 Years of Accomplishment* (Bangalore: National Tuberculosis Institute, 2000), 3.

4 Brimnes, N. (2016) Languished Hopes: Tuberculosis, the State and International Assistance in Twentieth-century India. Hyderabad, Orient Blackswan, pp. 229–232.

5 Tuberculosis chemotherapy Centre, Madras, 'A concurrent comparison of home and sanatorium treatment of pulmonary tuberculosis in South India', *Bulletin of the world Health Organization*, 21, 1959, 51–144.

6 C.V. Ramakrishnan et al., 'The role of diet in the treatment of tuberculosis', *Bulletin of the world Health Organization*, 25, 1961, 339–359, on p. 357.

7 Interview with Debabar Banerji, 4. February 2014; D. Banerji, 'A social science approach to strengthening India's national tuberculosis programme', *Indian Journal of Tuberculosis*, 40, 1993, 61–82 on p. 64. D. Banerji, *The Making of a Community Health Physician in India. An Intellectual Autobiography* (New Delhi: Lok Prakash, 2017), 38–39, 46. The difference between approach taken by the Tuberculosis Chemotherapy Centre and by the NTI, and the tensions it created, is convincingly analysed in S.S. Amrith, 'In search of a "magic bullet" for tuberculosis: South India and beyond, 1955–65', *Social History of Medicine*, 17 (1), 2004, 113–130, particularly pp. 122–127. See also Brimnes, *Languished Hopes*, 185–189, 192–193.

8 P.V. Benjamin, *Tuberculosis in India* (New Delhi: Ministry of Health, 1961), 28.

9 Banerji, 'A Social Science approach', 64. See also Banerji, *The Making of a Community Health Physician*, 37–48. On Mahler's years in India, see N. Brimnes, 'Negotiating social medicine in a post-colonial context: Halfdan Mahler in India 1951–61', *Medical History*, 67 (1), 2023, 5–22, doi:10.1017/mdh.2023.11.

10 Brimnes, *Languished Hopes*, 224–226. The Andersen quote is from Stig Andersen, 'Assignment Report on National Tuberculosis Institute, India', 21. November 1963, 17. SEA/TB/49, WHO Archives, Geneva.

11 Brimnes, *Languished Hopes*, 226–227. Quotes from 'Recommendations for a district tuberculosis control programme [1962]', 5 in WHO-IND-MBD-003, 1958–1969, and M. Piot, 'Outline of a district tuberculosis programme', *Indian Journal of Tuberculosis*, 9 (3), 1962, 151–156 on p. 153. Piot's article also contained a slightly different version of the calculation of the cost of adding PAS to the standard regimen.

12 'Chemotherapy and Chemoprophylaxis in Tuberculosis Control. Report of a Study Group', *WHO Technical Report Series*, 141, 1957, 8–9.

13 Brimnes, *Languished Hopes*, 189–197, 228. S. Andersen and D. Banerji, 'A sociological inquiry into an urban tuberculosis control programme in India', *Bulletin of the WHO*, 29 (5), 1963, 685–700, on p. 686; Piot, 'Outline', 153.

14 W. Fox, 'The problem of self-administration of drugs; with particular reference to pulmonary tuberculosis', *Tubercle* (London) 39, 1958, 269–274, on p. 273. The article was based on a report to the WHO Study Group that phrased the pertinent questions quoted above. Fox later changed his view and looked more towards organizational issues. See Brimnes, *Languished Hopes*, 193–194.

15 Andersen and Banerji, 'A sociological inquiry', 691, 698. This was also the message taken away by the (unidentified) authors of the Introduction to this particular volume of the *Bulletin*: Andersen's and Banerji's work had "brought to light the fact that the major weaknesses of the programme lay, not in the less than ideal drug regimen (isoniazid alone) prescribed, nor even in the failure of some patients to complete the course of treatment, bit in basic shortcomings in administration and organization". See 'Introduction', 559–63, on p. 561.

16 Eventually, BCG vaccination was 'integrated' into the 'Expanded programme of immunization from 1974'. Brimnes, *Languished Hopes*, 229–232, 263. Quotes from H. Mahler, 'Final Report on India BCG', [1955]; http://www.cf-hst.net/UNICEF-TEMP/Doc-Repository/doc/doc450078.PDF and S. Andersen, 'India 103 – National Tuberculosis Programme', Quartey Field Report, 1st Quarter 1961, 3 April, 3, NTI Library, Bangalore. For the 1962 position, see 'Recommendations for a district tuberculosis control programme [1962]', 7 in WHO-IND-MBD-003, 1958–69, WHO Archives, Geneva.

17 'Recommendations for a district tuberculosis control programme [1962]', 5.

18 'Expert Committee on Tuberculosis: Eighth Report', *WHO Technical Reports Series*, 290, 1964. Quotes from pp. 13, 17.

19 Brimnes, *Languished Hopes*, 221–223, 250–251. In 1993 Banerji stated that 378 out of India's 438 districts had 'implemented' the NTP. This would amount to a coverage 87% at district level. See Banerji, 'A social Science Approach', 74.

20 Brimnes, *Languished Hopes*, 223, 251–252.

21 Brimnes, *Languished Hopes*, 226–227; 255–257. In an interview given in 2014, Banerji maintained that monotherapy with isoniazid was rare in the NTP. Banerji, interview 2014. Quote from N.L. Bordia, 'National tuberculosis programme', *Indian Journal of Tuberculosis*, 14 (4), 1967, 183–185, on p. 185.

22 A programme review conducted in 1988 reported compliance rates between 25.7% and 26.8% for the period 1984–1986. See Institute of Communication, Operations Research and Community Involvement (ICORCI), 'In Depth Study on National Tuberculosis Programme of India', Bangalore: ICORCI, 1988, 33. See also Brimnes, *Languished Hopes*, 228, 257.

23 Brimnes, *Languished Hopes*, 257–258.

24 Brimnes, *Languished Hopes*, 264. I have only had access to an incomplete copy of this review.

25 See Institute of Communication, Operations Research and Community Involvement (ICORCI), 'In Depth Study on National Tuberculosis Programme of India', Bangalore: ICORCI, 1988, 24–26, 216. Quoted from p. 219.

26 See Institute of Communication, Operations Research and Community Involvement (ICORCI), 'In Depth Study on National Tuberculosis Programme of India', Bangalore: ICORCI, 1988, 211–214.

27 See Institute of Communication, Operations Research and Community Involvement (ICORCI), 'In Depth Study on National Tuberculosis Programme of India', Bangalore: ICORCI, 1988, 45, 135–139, 200.

28 See Institute of Communication, Operations Research and Community Involvement (ICORCI), 'In Depth Study on National Tuberculosis Programme of India', Bangalore: ICORCI, 1988, 3.

29 See Institute of Communication, Operations Research and Community Involvement (ICORCI), 'In Depth Study on National Tuberculosis Programme of India', Bangalore: ICORCI, 1988, 56, 113–117.

30 See Institute of Communication, Operations Research and Community Involvement (ICORCI), 'In Depth Study on National Tuberculosis Programme of India', Bangalore: ICORCI, 1988, 56, 190.

31 See Institute of Communication, Operations Research and Community Involvement (ICORCI), 'In Depth Study on National Tuberculosis Programme of India', Bangalore: ICORCI, 1988, 19, 216.

32 'Tuberculosis Programme Review, India. September 1992', WHO /TB/95.186. Copy in NTI, Library, Bangalore, 4–5, 19–20.

33 'Tuberculosis Programme Review', 4–5, 25.

34 See Institute of Communication, Operations Research and Community Involvement (ICORCI), 'In Depth Study on National Tuberculosis Programme of India', Bangalore: ICORCI, 1988, 119, 218; 'Tuberculosis Programme Review', 4, 23, 53.

35 'Tuberculosis Programme Review', 13.

36 'Tuberculosis Programme Review', 9, 13, 25.

37 'Tuberculosis Programme Review', 35.

38 Christolph Gradmann, 'Treatment on trial: Tanzania's national programme, the international union against tuberculosis and lung disease, and the road to DOTS, 1977–1991', *Journal of the History of Medicine and Allied Sciences*, 74 (3), 2019, 316–343, quoted from p. 328. This article is the main source for my account of the Tanzanian programme, but see also J.-P. Gaudillière, C. Gradmann and A. McDowell, 'The not so distant past, tuberculosis and the DOTS challenge', in J.-P. Gaudillière et al. (eds.) *Global Health*, 2020, 52–80, pp. 61–66.

39 Gradmann, 'Treatment on Trial', 326–327, 329–330, 338. The SCCs often included streptomycin, which had to be injected. Hence the preference for initial hospitalization.

40 World Bank, *Investing in Health. World Development Report 1993*, World Bank, 1993, 17.

41 World Bank, *Investing in Health. World Development Report 1993*, World Bank, 1993, 10, 36, 63. See in particular the figure on p. 62, in which 'Chemotherapy for tuberculosis' yields more DALYs than any other intervention for only moderate costs.

42 N. Chorev, *The World Health Organization Between North and South* (Ithaca: Rutgers University Press, 2012), 124–159.

43 A. Kochi, 'The global tuberculosis situation and the new control strategy of the World Health Organization', *Tubercle*, 72, 1991, 1–6.

44 World Health organization, 'TB – a global Emergency', 1994, 2, 6, 7.

45 The acronym DOTS was given to the strategy a year later, in 1995. Gaudillière, Gradmann and Mc Dowell, 'The not so distant past', 52. For the elements in DOTS,

see 'What is DOTS. A guide to Understanding the WHO-recommended TB control strategy known as DOTS', *WHO*, 1999, 8; Beaudevin et al., 'Global health and the new world order', 9.

46 *A Brief History of Tuberculosis Control in India*, Geneva. WHO, 2010, 3.

47 Banerji, 'A social science approach', 61–68, quotes from pp. 61, 66 and 68. Banerji here referred to the oration given by Mahler, at the 'silver jubilee' of NTI in 1985.

48 D. Baenrji, *Serious Implications of the Proposed Revised National Tuberculosis Control Programme for India* (New Delhi: Voluntary Health Association of India, 1997), 3, 12–14, 21, quotes from pp. 14 and 21.

49 Banerji, *Serious Implications*, 38. For timely what he terms 'Banerji's nostalgia', See Gaudillière, Gradmann and McDowell, 'The not so distant past', 70–74.

50 Banerji, *Serious Implications*. In various form the allegation that tuberculosis was in natural decline is found on pp. 6, 8, 28, 35, 45, 49. Final quote on p. 9.

51 Banerji, *Serious Implications*, 5, 28, 32. Quote form p. 28. Grzybowsky had visited India as WHO consultant with Karel Styblo in 1971.

52 Banerji's intervention led to a meeting between representatives of the concerned NGOs (including Banerji), the World Bank and WHO. The disagreements persisted. Banerji, 'Serious Implications', 86–97.

53 Engel, 'Standardization and localization', 34–40; Jens Seeberg, 'The event of DOTS and the transformation of the tuberculosis syndemic in India', *Cambridge Anthropology*, 32 (1), 2014, 95–113.

# 5 Tuberculosis, community engagement, and person-centred care in Bangladesh

## Successes and challenges

*Shahaduz Zaman and Mahfuza Rifat*

## Introduction

Being the youngest country in South Asia,[1] Bangladesh had many challenges related to social, economic, political, cultural, and environmental development from the beginning. Despite all the challenges, however, Bangladesh has made remarkable strides in reducing poverty and instigating development processes over the past five decades. According to the World Bank (2024), the country is one of the fastest-growing economies in Asia. Further, Bangladesh ranks second in Asia in terms of gender parity with women as head of state, opposition party leader, and speaker of the parliament. Regardless of achieving notable progress on most health indicators for the Sustainable Development Goals (SDGs), Bangladesh continues to suffer from high prevalence of diarrheal diseases, tuberculosis (TB), dengue, and many other communicable or infectious diseases (Houben and Dodd 2016; Salje et al. 2019).

The Bangladesh war or the Liberation War of 1971 damaged the infrastructure and institutions in the country at a catastrophic level, which caused developmental challenges and dire poverty. Weak economic infrastructure, inadequate human capital, fragile institutions of education, health, and development were common features of Bangladesh in its early days (Ibrahim 2017). In 1972, the Bangladeshi population that was living below the poverty line was estimated as 90% (World Bank 2024). According to Ibrahim (2017), Bangladesh had an illiteracy rate around 80% in the early 1970s. Various government and non-governmental policies played a crucial role in overcoming these challenges and achieving human development outcomes (Asadullah 2018). The Female Secondary School Assistance Programme (FSSAP), BRAC's Education Programme (BEP), and Female Stipend Programme (FSP) all played significant roles in improving the literacy rate of the population, and also improving the living conditions of people, including

DOI: 10.4324/9781032634647-5

their health status (Rust 2016). By 2021, the literacy rate of Bangladesh improved from 20% in the early 1970s to 75.6% (New Age 2021). The Government of Bangladesh managed to establish a remarkable relationship with its home-grown civil society organizations such as Gonoshasthaya Kendra (or People's Health Center), Grameen Bank, Bangladesh Rural Advancement Committee (BRAC), and the Association for Social Advancement (ASA) from the beginning. According to Baser and Hasnath (2022), the civil society organizations in Bangladesh have been delivering services for poor communities in both urban and rural on the following five categories.

1 Poverty alleviation and socioeconomic development.
2 Nonformal education and skills development.
3 Healthcare services and advocacy.
4 Environmental services, education, and advocacy.
5 Promoting human rights.

The home-gown NGOs are not only playing a key role in development and humanitarian work in Bangladesh, but also in responding to disaster and development challenges in other countries in the world. For example, BRAC has been responding to disasters and development challenges in more than 12 countries in Asia and Africa (BRAC 2024). The NGO is currently considered to be the largest NGO in the world (Ravelo 2021). Founded in Bangladesh in 1972, BRAC grew to become an international development and humanitarian NGO that partners with over 100 million people living with inequality and poverty.

In this backdrop, this chapter examines the community engagement and person-centred care interventions in Bangladesh in relation to dealing with TB.

## Method and approach

A review of published literature and documents was conducted with key focus on TB control, community-based care, and health system. This chapter documents the changes in adopting new strategies of the TB programme and the context of community-based care over the period of three decades. This changed after adoption of World Health Organisation's (WHO) recommended Directly Observed Treatment, Short-course (DOTS) strategy.[2] According to WHO, the best method to cure TB is known as DOTS, which is a cost-effective way to stop the spreading of TB in communities (WHO 1996).

DOTS has five main components (WHO 1999):

1 Government commitment (including political will at all levels, and establishment of a centralized and prioritized system of TB monitoring, recording, and training)
2 Case detection by sputum smear microscopy

3   Standardized treatment regimen directly of six to nine months observed by a healthcare worker or community health worker for at least the first two months
4   Drug supply
5   A standardized recording and reporting system that allows assessment of treatment results

The authors included key community engagement examples in Bangladesh which included community volunteers, informal providers, and community clinic-level staff supported by the government. Both the authors have been closely involved in the TB control programme in Bangladesh in different capacities including designing, delivering, monitoring, and evaluation of interventions. In this, these experiences were critically examined within the social, political, cultural, economic, and environmental context of Bangladesh. Within this critical analysis, the positionalities of the authors had a vital advantage. Both the authors are from Bangladesh. The first author of this chapter has an interdisciplinary background with more than 15 years of experience in conducting research in global public health. In Bangladesh, he has been closely engaging with various NGOs, including BRAC. The second author of this chapter is a public health specialist with research experiences in public health, health systems, TB, nutrition, infectious diseases, and epidemiology.

In this background, the authors took an approach to tease out the successes and failures of community engagement, and person-centred care interventions in relation to TB in Bangladesh. This is somewhat a success story, however, there are many areas to be improved.

## Locating TB in Bangladeshi context

According to the WHO regional divisions, Bangladesh is located in Southeast Asia, and has been listed under the high TB burden countries for TB and drug-resistant tuberculosis (DR-TB) (WHO 2023).[3] With a current incidence of estimated 221 per 100,000 population, as many as 0.26 million people affected by TB received treatment by the national TB control programme (NTP) and partner organizations, in 2022 (WHO 2023). Mortality of TB has been reduced remarkably to 36% since 1990. The treatment success rate has been sustained to more than 90% in the country over decades. A main feature of TB management in Bangladesh which contributed to better treatment outcome has been the partnership approach of Government, NGOs, and communities complementing each other in the resource-limited setting (NTP 2023). Community engagement through different approaches has been observed to contribute towards positive treatment outcomes. Over the period of three decades, diagnostic, treatment, and prevention modalities have been changed with new advancement, globally and nationally in Bangladesh.

Initial efforts of countrywide TB service coverage, known as DOTS coverage, were expanded through diagnosis through microscopy followed by integrated management of TB in primary healthcare model (NTP 2023). Shifting the diagnostic approach to molecular technologies, mainly Gene expert, also underwent countrywide expansion in the current decade as the newer recommended method for TB diagnosis. Recent advancements in tuberculosis (TB) management include the introduction of newer drugs and shorter treatment regimens, particularly for drug-resistant TB (DR-TB). Additionally, TB preventive therapy has been incorporated to enhance control efforts. Community-based care models, including Directly Observed Treatment (DOT), are evolving towards more person-centered approaches, focusing on individualized care for patients. Moreover, Bangladesh has evolved towards becoming a lower-middle-income country and aspires to become the middle-income country status through economic and social changes over the coming decades (Sen 2013). In this paper, we reviewed community-based care for TB management in the context of changed scenarios including TB diagnostic and treatment modality, along with the changed landscape of the country in terms of economic and social changes.

### TB in Bangladesh

In 2022, the world witnessed new reported TB reaching to 7.5 million, which surpassed the pre-COVID baseline and previous historical peak of 7.1 million in 2019 (WHO 2023). Alongside, TB caused an estimated 1.30 million deaths globally in the same year. The estimated TB incidence rate (new cases per 100,000 population per year) stood at 133 in 2022 underlining the widespread impact of this disease globally.

In 2022, the WHO regions of South-East Asia observed the highest incidence of TB cases, accounting for 46% of the total global cases. Thirty high TB burden countries accounted for 87% of the world's TB cases in 2022, and two-thirds of the global total was in eight countries including 3.6% from Bangladesh. The estimated incidence of TB per 100,000 is 221 in Bangladesh, with a mortality rate of 24 per 100,000 population (WHO 2023). TB has been reported to be the fifth cause of death in Bangladesh as per WHO Data, 2019. In 2022, the WHO estimated 379,000 (CI 273,000–493,000) people with TB in the country, and 42,000 (CI 27,000–61,000) people died of TB. The country notified a total of 262,731 people with TB in 2022. HIV positive TB incidence is 0.43% as HIV prevalence is low in Bangladesh. Proportion of drug resistance among new and previously treated patients are 1.1 and 5.5%, respectively (WHO 2023). The absolute number of estimated DR-TB is high considering the population of the country.

Since 2005, the number of TB cases notified in Bangladesh has been on a steady rise. The enhanced case-finding with the establishment and scale-up of the DOTS programme led to a rapid increase in bacteriologically confirmed pulmonary TB cases. A complete TB service coverage was achieved in all districts of Bangladesh by 2007. The rise in bacteriologically confirmed notifications in recent years has been contributed by the expanded utilization of GeneXpert diagnostics. A countrywide major expansion of this new technology took place from 2018 to 2020.

Although the incidence rate over time has not been decreased, death due to TB has been reduced remarkably to 36% from 2015 to 2022 (NTP 2023). Treatment success rate for drug-sensitive and drug-resistant TB (MDR/RR TB) has been high for years, observed as 97% and 73%, respectively (WHO 2023).

## Community-based service provision: Bringing the services to doorsteps

Community-based approach in healthcare provision has been a well adopted in Bangladesh since the birth of the country after liberation in 1971, mainly to address the shortage of human resources mainly to reach large populations, especially living in rural areas with limited resources (El Arifeen et al. 2013). Government and NGOs have undertaken capacity development activities for the community health workers and community stakeholders on many health issues including TB.

Since 1991, the National Tuberculosis Control Programme, operating under the Directorate General of Health Services, has established partnerships with NGOs through Memorandums of Understanding (MoUs) to implement the DOTS strategy. (NTP, 2023). Community-based approaches have been tried through these NGO partnerships. Community health volunteers such as BRAC's *Shasthya Shebika* (a woman who provides basic healthcare services in the community – or Community Health Workers)[4] and village doctor network of Damien Foundation served as primary point of contact for TB symptom identification, and referral for diagnosis. This group of community workers and informal providers trained on basic messages of TB, brought the treatment of TB close to the patient's home by ensuring directly observed treatment (El Arifeen et al. 2013). Bangladesh has seen a tremendous improvement in successful cure rates with the engagement of community health workers, village doctors, and cured TB patients in combating the disease. The series of events are implemented in collaboration with the national programme and non-governmental organizations.

In 1984, BRAC launched an experimental TB control programme in Bangladesh, employing community health workers for local detection and treatment. BRAC's Community Health Workers (*Shasthya Shebika*) selected from the community level reach out to the community and screen out individuals for basic TB symptoms, refer for diagnosis, transport samples to sputum collection centres, or at the laboratory. After diagnosis, *Shasthya Shebika* monitors the daily intake of TB medicine during the treatment period (4, 5). Community members diagnosed with TB are provided with directly observed therapy at the community level in proximity of the DOT provider. This initiative supplemented the national TB control efforts and showed promising results in improving treatment success rate (Chowdhury et al. 1997). *Shasthya Shebika* received financial incentive of around 8 USD to complete monitoring of each drug-sensitive TB patient. They also receive nominal earnings from selling other non-TB common health products supported under BRAC. The BRAC trained and expanded the number of *Shasthya Shebika* to 43,000 by 2020 (Perry 2020).

Bangladesh with a large private healthcare sector present in both rural and urban areas that encompasses both formal and informal individual practitioners, as well as private commercial and voluntary institutions (Ahmed et al. 2013). The informal healthcare providers comprise the largest segment of the health sector workforce that play a crucial role in delivering healthcare services in Bangladesh (Hamid et al. 2006). The estimated total density of unrecognized and unqualified health workers including informal health workers was 15.84 per 10,000 population in 2019 (Ministry of Health and Family Welfare Bangladesh 2021). Among them semi-qualified allopathic providers such as community health workers, medical assistants, and trained midwives, unqualified allopathic providers including drug shop retailers, rural doctors, traditional healers (practitioners of Ayurvedic, Unani, and homeopathic medicine), and faith healers are also included (WHO 2015). Studies suggest that about 75% of the rural and 84% of the urban population depend on private, small, informal healthcare service providers who are mostly semi-skilled with no professional training (WHO 2015). In Bangladesh, 13% of treatment-seekers use government services, 27% use private/NGO services, and 60% use unqualified services (Cockcroft et al. 2004; Ministry of Health and Family Welfare Bangladesh 2023).

Although public sector and NGO services are accessible, many individuals opt for assistance from drug shop retailers and village doctors for common health issues. The Damien Foundation acknowledged the widespread utilization of informal providers, mainly drug shop retailers, some of them have some training as rural doctors (non-graduate informal), engaged particularly in the impoverished rural population, due to their proximity and affordability in the community. A network of patient friendly Directly Observed Treatment (DOT) services has been established at the community level through the voluntary involvement of informal providers, cured patients, and local opinion leaders. At present around 10,000 fixed DOT Providers are involved in providing DOT in the area covered by Damien Foundation (Damien Foundation 2022). Informal providers trained on basic messages of TB, brought the treatment of TB close to patients home by ensuring directly observed treatment. Proximity to community positioned them well to detect TB symptoms and monitor treatment, refer TB presumptive for diagnosis to designated TB centre and act as a local treatment supporter. Bangladesh policy does not allow informal providers to initiate treatment, they can only monitor the treatment intake once diagnosed at health facility level by registered physician. This partnership with the informal providers, especially village doctors, has been recognized as a Public Private Mix (PPM) approach by WHO (WHO 2011). Despite the absence of financial incentive, the main motivation of village doctors is the social recognition and trust of the community that they gain through positive results of TB treatment monitoring. Informal providers consider their role as DOT provider as an opportunity to provide high-quality, free-of-cost TB medicine care to society, which may in turn support their business indirectly by increasing clients at their premises. Many of them also consider it a moral responsibility to society (Hamid et al. 2006). Community health workers have been posing as the frontline workers in active case finding for decades in rural communities. The early case detection of the disease is equally important, as it is to ensure the treatment completion of the patient to avoid the development of drug resistance (Garg et al. 2020; Myburgh et al. 2023).

With steadfast dedication, community health workers visit TB patients at home, providing reassurance and ensuring prompt sample collection for accurate diagnosis and timely intervention. Community health workers educate communities on TB symptoms, transmission, and prevention, emphasizing prompt medical care. They actively search for symptomatic individuals, conduct screenings, and refer cases for diagnosis and treatment, aiding early identification. They also help trace contacts for screening, thereby facilitating the implementation of TB Preventive Therapy (TPT). Overall, they facilitate seamless community-healthcare facility linkage for comprehensive TB management. Their support extends beyond households to health clinics, ensuring patients never face TB alone. These CHWs, at the core of every community, tirelessly combat TB, exemplifying the power of compassion and community action in the fight against the disease. The engagement of CHWs, village doctors, and cured TB patients at community level is a cost-effective intervention, and they must be empowered to ensure universal access to essential services and seamless referrals to higher-level care.

Community-based care under the public healthcare services is managed through the domiciliary healthcare provider and community clinics. Bangladesh established community clinics for around 6,000 rural population and more than 13,000 community clinics are currently functional (Riaz et al. 2020). A community healthcare provider (CHCP) along with a health assistant (HA) and a family welfare assistant (FWA) supports community-based care under the public system and covers a broad range of services including maternal health, nutrition, communicable and non-communicable through screening, basic management, and referral (Joarder et al. 2019).

These community clinic structures are revolutionary approach in Bangladesh to bring health care further close to the community and its inbuilt sustainable structure. Community clinic staff are also engaged in TB screening and referral. Community clinic staff identify the people with TB symptoms and refer them for diagnosis to the health facility at the subdistrict level.

Community clinic staff and TB-NGO partners organize sputum collection camp at community clinics for TB diagnosis. In addition, field-level staff, including family welfare assistant (FWA) and health assistants (HA), also identify TB presumptive at household level during their regular health-related visit. Unlike the NGO-supported community workers who receive incentive for services, community clinic staff are salaried staff paid by the government budget (Perry 2020).

## Acceptability, appropriateness, and feasibility of community approaches within recent context

Despite the successful implementation for decades, community-based care in TB faces challenges with the changed circumstances that evolved through ongoing development such as urbanization, availability of choices for services due to improved road network, digitalization, and improved economic status. However, access is not always beneficial due to large unregulated private health care. Community health workers may not always be the first contact of people in this changing environment and their role may need to be shifted from service provision to referral (El Arifeen et al. 2013).

Key motivating factors for effective participation in the TB programme by the community health workers and informal providers were mainly recognition, access to free training and knowledge updates, confidence from being entrusted with TB drugs, subsequent social respect, and credibility in the community, which is also observed in other settings (Colvin et al. 2021; Dam et al. 2022). Additionally, *Sashthya Shebika* receives incentive for completing the Directly Observed Treatment (DOT). Incentive mechanisms varied among the community-level providers (WHO 2020). The relevance of similar incentives, or no incentive at all, may not be as motivating a factor as it used to be in the past. Alternative economic opportunities may divert their role from previous social interest focused role which is more profound in urban areas. Emerging needs of addressing the dual burden of communicable and non-communicable diseases and relevant capacity development were also observed as community-level requirement. Volunteer effort, or low-cost services provided through community health workers by considering "recognition" as only motivating factor, may not be as relevant in the changing context.

However, during the COVID-19 pandemic, the importance of community engagement, role of community, and informal providers received further attention and emphasis (Ballard et al. 2020). People with other diseases including TB also suffered during the initial period of pandemic, affected by movement restriction events to reduce the transmission of COVID-19. The shift from facility level care and need for community level care reemerged to manage TB and other diseases during the COVID-19 pandemic years (Zimmer et al. 2021).

## Transition in TB management modalities and readiness of community approach

Sputum smear microscopy, a 100-year-old technology for TB diagnosis, had been widely used in low and middle-income countries and being replaced by the rapid molecular technologies. Rapid molecular methods detect mycobacterial antigens or DNA. These tools can also detect the resistance to anti-TB medicines (Steingart 2021).

Bangladesh has also adopted new molecular technologies recommended by WHO and gradually expanded in the country, which is mostly Gene Xpert, and very recently Truenat at limited scale. These tests also can detect the resistance pattern of TB bacteria at the same time and have reduced the long duration of diagnosis of DR-TB. Rapid molecular tests are being used to detect first-line and second-line resistance of TB which is also under expansion in Bangladesh (NTP 2023).

Bangladesh follows the latest WHO guideline of six-month TB treatment for drug susceptible. Bangladesh also adopted the Short all Oral TB Regimen (SOTR) since 2020 and under process to adopt BPaL (bee-pal) regimen (comprised of bedaquiline, pretomanid, and linezolid) for DR-TB. These newer regimens replaced the previously used longer regimen for DR-TB treatment. Damien Foundation in Bangladesh also tried the shorter regimen for DR-TB treatment which has shown path towards adopting a shorter regimen for DR-TB patients and importance of research in this area. The previous long hospitalization period has been replaced by ambulatory treatment of DR-TB.

Community component as an integral part of TB care had to adapt with necessary changes in the TB strategy over time which included capacity development of community workers and community-based providers in Bangladesh as well as other settings (Das et al. 2019). The changes took place along the newer technologies and TB management approaches which have been taking place in the country over decades. Role of community-based providers included but not limited to- referral of patient, sample transportation for molecular testing, treatment support at community level, monitoring, and referral for side effects.

Another new area of community engagement is TB preventive therapy where people with TB infections are provided with WHO-recommended TB preventive therapy. According to Bangladesh NTP guideline, primarily household contacts will receive TPT after a screening process. Community engagement is crucial for TB preventive therapy implementation as it includes household contact investigation, counselling healthy household members to participate in screening, and take medicine for prevention of TB. Implementing TB preventive therapy without community engagement is hardly feasible and justifies the importance of community-based care in TB in recent eras.

## Directly observed treatment (DOT) for TB and patient centred care

Directly observed treatment for TB was introduced to ensure the regular intake of anti-TB medicines under supervision of a trained health worker which has been a major role of the community health workers in Bangladesh and was strongly recommended by the TB treatment guideline. The recent approach of "patient centered care" emphasizes patient's convenience, choice, and rights (WHO 2019; Myburgh et al. 2023; Stillo 2024). Patient organizations often consider DOT as a binding over choices (Adams et al. 2013; Mhimbira et al. 2016). Both approaches, DOT and patient centred care do not conflict with each other if the community-based care can understand the needs and choice of the patient, ensures confidentiality to avoid possible stigma.

The WHO recommended Directly Observed Therapy, Short Course (DOTS) strategy during 1990s which included directly observed treatment approach for TB along with other components, including political commitment, TB detection, uninterrupted supplies, and impact measurement. Considering the duration TB treatment period, which is currently six-months for drug sensitive TB, irregular intake of anti-TB medicine may lead to treatment failure and drug resistance. Supervised intake of medicine reduces the risk of treatment interruption. People who received self-administered treatment showed lower success rate compared to the patients under DOT. Receiving every dose in front of a healthcare worker at facilities poses challenges to the patients considering travel time, distance, and cost. Community-based DOT replaces the facility-based DOT and improves access. The WHO also recommended community health workers, peer groups or family members can be engaged to support DOT. Civil society organization for TB urged for a shift from the facility-based DOT towards the patient-centred approaches. However, community-based DOT also possess limitations to address patient's perspective such as individual freedom, privacy, stigma which may affect their personal and work life (Zimmer et al. 2021). Civil society organizations that are working on TB emphasized patient centred approach and individual choices to decide who will observe the treatment. The DOT provided by the family members may not work for the people who do not have supportive environment or capacity in the family to perform DOT (Zimmer et al. 2021). Confidentiality is crucial to protect rural women from stigmatization, especially for younger women. Workers often do not want to disclose their TB status to the employer. Patient choice has been addressed this way in Bangladesh context as well. Recent developments in video-based and other digitally supported DOT innovations have also been tried on a limited scale in some settings. Community-based DOT keeps the potential to support TB treatment by emphasizing the patient's choice and freedom component in decision-making.

However, it is crucial to carefully consider the ongoing balance between individual freedoms and public health. Scholars have pointed out that there exists a fundamental conflict across all public health challenges, from infectious to chronic diseases, between the well-being of the community and that of the individual. Acknowledging these tough choices is essential when shaping policies (WHO 2019). This issue becomes even more significant in a collective society such as Bangladesh.

## Economic and social transition in Bangladesh and motivation of community workers

With a population of over 174 million, currently, Bangladesh is the 8th most populous country in the world. It is also among the most densely populated countries with a population density of about 1,342 people per square km throughout the country. The country is currently growing at an annual rate of around 1%. Life expectancy at birth currently stands at 72 years for males and 76 years for females (NIPORT 2023). About 59% of the population of Bangladesh were rural dwellers in 2023. Bangladesh, being one of the poorest nations at birth in 1971, reached lower-middle income status in 2015 as classified by the World Bank. Poverty declined from 11.8% in 2010 to 5.0% in 2022, based on the international poverty line of $2.15 a day (using 2017 Purchasing Power Parity exchange rate). Human development outcomes have been improved in many dimensions. Despite these gains, inequality exists and has slightly narrowed in rural areas and widened in urban areas. With the shifting economic status and existing disease prevalence in the country, Bangladesh continues to face challenges in combating TB. Factors such as population density, limited access to health care in remote areas, and socioeconomic disparities contribute to the persistence of TB. TB programme is funded by domestic and external funding sources. Government covers a substantial proportion including first-line drugs and health infrastructure and human resources for health supporting TB. TB medicine and diagnostic services are free for patients.

Community-based service for TB in the changed economic and social context seems challenging considering current economic and social changes and expansion of urbanization (El Arifeen et al. 2013). Compared to rural areas, community health concept was not applicable in urban settings. Household visits are often limited and acceptance of a similar status of a rural community provider is limited to urban population. Many working populations, especially in the urban slums of big cities, are not available during the daytime as people go out for work, which may require a different timing for community-based care. The changed economic status might have effect on motivating factors for the community health workers of rural areas as well. Although WHO recommended a financial package for the community health workers based on the role and engagement, approaches to incentive varies (Ballard et al. 2021; Gadsden et al. 2021; Ballard et al. 2022). Majorities of the community health workers receive the motivation of their work through social recognition, and trust of the community, some receive some direct or indirect financial incentives in Bangladesh for their engagement in TB and other health issues (Onazi et al. 2020). Sustainability of the incentive and the outcome are often debated. Although non-financial incentives are provided through skill development which motivates to continue their work, it is often difficult to maintain the same effort considering income level, availability of other opportunities, and competitive environment due to the presence of multiple providers within the current context (WHO 2018a; Colvin et al. 2021). Community health workers may accept other income-generating options over low-paid community work. Demand side change in receiving community care may be observed in increased access to treatment and change in the treatment need such as epidemiological transition to double burden of communicable and non-communicable diseases (El Arifeen et al. 2013). The presence of pluralistic healthcare system is not always positive being unregulated and affects the high out of pocket cost of the patients (Ahmed et al. 2013).

However, cultural norms of helping each other is a common practice in rural communities of Bangladesh which may sustain the practices of community-level care. The need for community-based care is well recognized in the emerging areas of TB management including active case finding (ACF) for TB, TB preventive therapy and contact screening, ambulatory care support, and reaching the last miles of ending TB (WHO 2018b; WHO 2019).

## Conclusion

Bangladesh has been an example of engaging community workers in health since the birth of the country. Engaging the rural women as community health volunteers, referral linkage with informal providers, and other community-level workers in TB, is well recognized. In Bangladesh, community engagement in TB is not a standalone strategy, it is supported by a network of field-level workers and managed through well-established health structures supported by Government and NGOs. These field workers also represent the community and work closely with the community and community-based providers through supportive supervision and capacity development. Sustainability of community-based care depends on the sustainability of total package of care.

Despite the challenges of changed socio-economic context, urbanization, technological advances, and access to multiple providers, community-based approaches in TB helped to maintain a high treatment success in the country, supported in early detection and helped the patients through patient-centred approach. Recent advances in TB diagnosis, including molecular technologies, are supported by a community-based referral network that facilitates the identification and referral of individuals with presumptive TB. Community-level support plays an important role in TB preventive therapy along with diagnosis and treatment support. Although community engagement evolved as a solution in resource-limited settings, high-income countries also used community health approaches to bridge the gap between facility and the community. In

Bangladesh, community-level treatment support for TB found to be effective. Patient choice and rights need to be addressed as the core of community engagement in TB acknowledging the tension between individual choice and collective.

When it comes to its own commitment and determination, Bangladesh has been an example to its South Asian neighbours. Similar to India and Papua New Guinea that we discuss in this book, Bangladesh has all the necessary social, political, cultural, economic, and environmental challenges that could prevent them from successfully conducting interventions on communicable diseases, including TB. However, the Bangladesh story has something to teach other low-and middle-income countries. First, there is a political commitment at the government level, which includes the willingness to collaborate with Non-Governmental Organisations (NGOs). Second, the NGOs in Bangladesh, especially the home-grown organizations such as BRAC is taking their learning seriously, and there is a long-term commitment to poor communities. This commitment is not just to respond to communicable diseases, however, to improve the lives of people through various development and educational activities. Finally, the Government of Bangladesh, NGOs, and higher education institutions are conducting serious monitoring and evaluation of these communicable disease interventions. Combining these with the Bangladesh aspiration to become a middle-income country pushes the prevention and cure of communicable diseases including TB.

## Acknowledgement

We extend our gratitude to Kazi Mariam Naher, Programme Specialist at the Damien Foundation, for her valuable assistance in drafting initial segments of this article.

## Notes

1 Although Bangladesh is a country in South Asia, according to the World Health Organisation's (WHO) regional divisions, Bangladesh belongs to Southeast Asia (SEA) region.

2 DOTS, also known as TB-DOTS. The technical strategy for DOTS was developed by Karel Styblo of the International Union Against TB & Lung Disease in the 1970s and 1980s, primarily in Tanzania, but also in Malawi, Nicaragua and Mozambique.

3 While taking the WHO regionalization, this chapter position Bangladesh as a South Asian country, which has similar social, political, cultural, economic, and environmental challenges as the other South Asian neighbours, including the impacts of colonization, and coloniality.

4 BRAC first adopted the Barefoot Doctor approach used in China a half-century ago and trained male paramedics, but then shifted the approach in the early 1980s to focus on women with lesser training who were often illiterate. They receive four weeks of basic training by the local BRAC office. They are trained to treat common medical conditions, to promote a wide variety of health behaviours, and to refer patients to preventive and curative services as appropriate.

# References

Adams, A.M., Ahmed, T., El Arifeen, S., Evans, T.G., Huda, T. and Reichenbach, L. (2013) Innovation for universal health coverage in Bangladesh: a call to action. *The Lancet*, 382(9910), 2104–2111.

Ahmed, S.M., Evans, T.G., Standing, H. and Mahmud, S. (2013) Harnessing pluralism for better health in Bangladesh. *The Lancet*, 382(9906), 1746–1755.

Asadullah, N., Trannoy, A., Tubeuf, S. and Yalonetzky, G. (2018) Fair and unfair educational inequality in a developing country: the role of pupil's effort. *ECINEQ: Society for the Study of Economic Inequality*, Working Paper Series, Rome, Italy. (No. 474).

Ballard, M., Bancroft, E., Nesbit, J., Johnson, A., Holeman, I., Foth, J., Rogers, D., Yang, J., Nardella, J., Olsen, H. and Raghavan, M. (2020) Prioritising the role of community health workers in the COVID-19 response. *BMJ Global Health*, 5(6), e002550.

Ballard, M., Odera, M., Bhatt, S., Geoffrey, B., Westgate, C. and Johnson, A. (2022) Payment of community health workers. *The Lancet Global Health*, 10(9), e1242.

Ballard, M., Westgate, C., Alban, R., Choudhury, N., Adamjee, R., Schwarz, R., Bishop, J., McLaughlin, M., Flood, D., Finnegan, K. and Rogers, A. (2021) Compensation models for community health workers: comparison of legal frameworks across five countries. *Journal of Global Health*, 11.

Baser, S., and Hasnath, S.A. (2023) The rise and fall of the NGOs in Bangladesh: what does the future hold? In V. Bobek and T. Horvat (Eds.), *Global Perspectives on Non-Governmental Organizations*. London: IntechOpen, pp. 69–100.

BRAC. (2024) *Where We work?* Available at: https://www.brac.net/where-we-work, Retrieved on May 16, 2024.

Chowdhury, A.M.R., Chowdhury, S., Islam, M.N., Islam, A. and Vaughan, J.P. (1997) Control of tuberculosis by community health workers in Bangladesh. *The Lancet*, 350(9072), 169–172.

Cockcroft, A., Milne, D. and Andersson, N. (2004) Health and population sector programme: third service delivery survey. *Canadian Institute for Energy Training Canada and Ministry of Health and Family Welfare Bangladesh*, 5.

Colvin, C.J., Hodgins, S. and Perry, H.B. (2021) Community health workers at the dawn of a new era: 8. Incentives and remuneration. *Health Research Policy and Systems*, 19, 1–25.

Damien Foundation. (2022) *Annual Report: 2022*. Dhaka: Damien Foundation.

Das, M., Pasupuleti, D., Rao, S., Sloan, S., Mansoor, H., Kalon, S., Hossain, F.N., Ferlazzo, G. and Isaakidis, P. (2019) GeneXpert and community health workers supported patient tracing for tuberculosis diagnosis in conflict-affected border areas in India. *Tropical Medicine and Infectious Disease*, 5(1), 1.

El Arifeen, S., Christou, A., Reichenbach, L., Osman, F.A., Azad, K., Islam, K.S., Ahmed, F., Perry, H.B. and Peters, D.H. (2013) Community-based approaches and partnerships: innovations in health-service delivery in Bangladesh. *The Lancet*, 382(9909), 2012–2026.

Gadsden, T., Mabunda, S.A., Palagyi, A., Maharani, A., Sujarwoto, S., Baddeley, M. and Jan, S. (2021) Performance-based incentives and community health workers' outputs, a systematic review. *Bulletin of the World Health Organization*, 99(11), 805.

Garg, T., Bhardwaj, M. and Deo, S. (2020) Role of community health workers in improving cost efficiency in an active case finding tuberculosis programme: an operational research study from rural Bihar, India. *BMJ Open*, 10(10), e036625.

Hamid Salim, M.A., Uplekar, M., Daru, P., Aung, M., Declercq, E. and Lönnroth, K. (2006) Turning liabilities into resources: informal village doctors and tuberculosis control in Bangladesh. *Bulletin of the World Health Organization*, 84(6), 479–484.

Houben, R.M. and Dodd, P.J. (2016) The global burden of latent tuberculosis infection: a re-estimation using mathematical modelling. *PLoS Medicine*, 13(10), e1002152.

Ibrahim, A. (2017) Re-thinking 'Poverty' in Bangladesh. *The Daily Star*. Available at: https://www.thedailystar.net/star-weekend/rethinking-poverty-bangladesh-1462156, Retrieved on May 16, 2024.

Joarder, T., Chaudhury, T.Z. and Mannan, I., 2019. Universal health coverage in Bangladesh: activities, challenges, and suggestions. *Advances in Public Health, 2019*(1), p.4954095

Mhimbira, F., Hella, J., Maroa, T., Kisandu, S., Chiryamkubi, M., Said, K., Mhalu, G., Mkopi, A., Mutayoba, B., Reither, K. and Gagneux, S. (2016) Home-based and facility-based directly observed therapy of tuberculosis treatment under programmatic conditions in urban Tanzania. *PLoS One*, 11(8), e0161171.

Ministry of Health and Family Welfare Bangladesh. (2021) *Assessment of Healthcare Providers in Bangladesh: 2021*. Dhaka: Ministry of Health and Family Welfare Bangladesh.

Ministry of Health and Family Welfare Bangladesh. (2023) *Bangladesh Health Workforce Strategy: 2023*. Dhaka: Ministry of Health and Family Welfare Bangladesh.

Myburgh, H., Baloyi, D., Loveday, M., Meehan, S.A., Osman, M., Wademan, D., Hesseling, A. and Hoddinott, G. (2023) A scoping review of patient-centred tuberculosis care interventions: gaps and opportunities. *PLOS Global Public Health*, 3(2), e0001357.

National Tuberculosis Control Programme (NTP). (2023) *National Strategic Plan to End Tuberculosis in Bangladesh 2024 to 2030*. Dhaka: Ministry of Health and Family Welfare.

New Age. (2021) *Bangladesh to Observe Int'l Literacy Day Today with 24.4pc of People Illiterate*. New Age: Bangladesh. Available at: https://www.newagebd.net/article/148506/bangladesh-to-observe-intl-literacy-day-today-with-244pc-of-people-illiterate, accessed on May 16, 2024.

NIPORT. (2023) *Bangladesh Demographic and Health Survey Report: 2023*. Dhaka: National Institute of Population Research and Training.

Onazi, O., Adejumo, A.O., Redwood, L., Okorie, O., Lawal, O., Azuogu, B., Gidado, M., Daniel, O.J. and Mitchell, E.M. (2020) Community health care workers in pursuit of TB: discourses and dilemmas. *Social Science & Medicine*, 246, 112756.

Perry, H., (ed). (2020) *Health for the People: National Community Health Worker Programs from Afghanistan to Zimbabwe*. Baltimore: The Maternal and Child Survival Program (MCSP).

Ravelo, J.L. (2021) *The World's Largest NGO Rethinks Its Future*, devex. Available at: https://www.devex.com/news/the-world-s-largest-ngo-rethinks-its-future-98629, accessed on May 16, 2024.

Riaz, B.K., Ali, L., Ahmad, S.A., Islam, M.Z., Ahmed, K.R. and Hossain, S. (2020) Community clinics in Bangladesh: a unique example of public-private partnership. *Heliyon*, 6(5) e03950.

Rust, P. (2016) Winning the war on illiteracy in Bangladesh. *BORGEN Magazine*. Available at: https://www.borgenmagazine.com/illiteracy-in-bangladesh/, accessed on May 16, 2024.

Salje, H., Paul, K.K., Paul, R., Rodriguez-Barraquer, I., Rahman, Z., Alam, M.S., Rahman, M., Al-Amin, H.M., Heffelfinger, J. and Gurley, E. (2019) Nationally-representative serostudy of dengue in Bangladesh allows generalizable disease burden estimates. *Elife*, 8, e42869.

Sen, A. (2013) What's happening in Bangladesh? *The Lancet*, 382(9909), 1966–1968.

Steingart, K. (2021) *WHO Consolidated Guidelines on Tuberculosis Module 3: Diagnosis-Rapid Diagnostics for Tuberculosis Detection*. Geneva: WHO.

Stillo, J. (2024) Connecting the DOTS: should we still be doing directly observed therapy? *Human Organization*, 83(1), 18–30.

WHO. (1996) *Tuberculosis*, WHO factsheet (revised). No. 104. Geneva: WHO.

WHO. (1999) *What Is DOTS?, A Guide to Understanding the WHO-Recommended TB Control Strategy Known as DOTS*. Geneva: WHO (WHO/CDS/CPC/TB/99.270).

WHO. (2011) *Regional Framework for Advocacy, Communication and Social Mobilization* (No. SEA-TB-333), WHO Regional Office for South-East Asia.

WHO. (2015) *Bangladesh Health System Review* (Vol. 5, No. 3), WHO Regional Office for the Western Pacific.

WHO. (2018a) *Baseline Assessment of Community-based TB Services in 8 WHO ENGAGE-TB Priority Countries*, (No. WHO/CDS/GTB/THC/18.34). Geneva: World Health Organization.

WHO. (2018b) *WHO Guideline on Health Policy and System Support to Optimize Community Health Worker Programmes*. Geneva: World Health Organization.

WHO. (2019) *People-Centred Framework for Tuberculosis Programme Planning and Prioritization: User Guide* (No. WHO/CDS/GTB/19.22). Geneva: World Health Organization.

WHO. (2020) *What Do We Know about Community Health Workers? A Systematic Review of Existing Reviews*. Geneva: World Health Organization.

WHO. (2023) *Global Tuberculosis Report: 2023*. Geneva: World Health Organization.

World Bank. (2024) *The World Bank in Bangladesh*. Available at: https://www.worldbank.org/en/country/bangladesh/overview#1, accessed on May 16, 2024.

Zimmer, A.J., Heitkamp, P., Malar, J., Dantas, C., O'Brien, K., Pandita, A. and Waite, R.C. (2021) Facility-based directly observed therapy (DOT) for tuberculosis during COVID-19: a community perspective. *Journal of Clinical Tuberculosis and Other Mycobacterial Diseases*, 24, 100248.

# 6 Communicable disease risk reduction – learning from the past

*Janaka Jayawickrama and*
*Arnab Chakraborty*

## Introduction

Based on the experiences from Papua New Guinea, India, and Bangladesh, this chapter delves into examining the usefulness of the idea of risk reduction. Particularly, for this chapter, we take this idea from the field of disasters. Stemming from the seminal article by O'Keefe et al. (1976), we define disasters when natural hazards collide with human systems. Years later to this article, in 2005, after the Hurricane Katrina, late Neil Smith provided an explanation that every stage of a natural hazard, including reasons, vulnerability, responses, and reconstruction, the human involvement increases or decreases risks. In that, we look at the idea of risk reduction from social, cultural, economic, political, and environmental perspectives, so that we could move the concept of disaster risk reduction to communicable disease risk reduction.

This chapter begins with defining risk reduction and takes through some examples and experiences from Cuba and Vietnam to explain how community-based disaster risk reduction works. Of course, for any risk reduction model to work effectively, there must be national-level political will and local-level community commitment. Both the examples from Cuba and Vietnam, this is visible. Then we introduce two more examples of communicable diseases and community-based approaches from Cuba and Sri Lanka. Through these learnings, we propose a communicable disease risk reduction framework that can be adapted in most contexts, especially in the Global South.

We invite the readers to be critical in reading this chapter. This is just a proposal. Bring your own experiences into understanding this proposal, and feel free to change and adapt what we a proposing.

## Defining risk reduction

Taking into consideration that single discipline analysis cannot solve real-world problems, this section critically engages with risk reduction literature, including concepts and practical approaches from the field of the study of disasters. Similar to communicable diseases, the human population has been

DOI: 10.4324/9781032634647-6

experiencing natural hazards such as floods, droughts, earthquakes, and land-slides from the beginning. The difference between communicable diseases and disasters is that bacteria and viruses cannot be seen by the human eye, however, disasters can be seen. In that, human beings have developed various strategies and approaches to dealing with disasters, especially to reduce risks of the impacts of such events.

The contemporary human civilization is experiencing the climate crisis, urban expansion and pressure, and technological hazards. The lack of disaster preparedness in various societies is increasingly transforming natural hazards causing disruptions to societies. While risks of disasters are rising, over the past 30 years, there have been increased discussions, and research on disaster risk reduction.

In terms of the United Nations system, disaster risk reduction (DRR) has become one of the most important agenda items. While the Sendai Framework for Disaster Risk Reduction (2015–2030) is the principal document for DRR, other global agendas including the Sustainable Development Goals (SDGs), the Paris Climate Agreement, the New Urban Agenda, and the Biodiversity Agenda have established targets that cannot be achieved without reducing the risks of disasters.

Table 6.1 presents the mainstream definitions that are emerging through the field of disaster studies:

The definitions in Table 6.1 by the United Nations Office for Disaster Risk Reduction (UNDRR) also provide a background to the idea of disaster risk reduction. According to the Sendai Framework for Disaster Risk Reduction (UNDRR 2015), disaster risk reduction can be defined as the prevention of new, and reduction of existing disaster risks, and managing residual risks. The UNDRR (2015) also argues that disaster risk reduction contributes to strengthening resilience of a society, and therefore facilitates the achievement of sustainable development.

## Community-based disaster risk reduction: Some examples

Communities have been responding to natural hazards even before the estab-lishment of states or organizations. The basic idea of community-based responses is based on family, relationships, and kinship, which is mainly to help each other. However, over the past 50 years, the disaster management community has developed this idea into organized format, so that the United Nations, governments, and organizations can engage with communities that are vulnerable to natural hazards in a systematic manner. In this book, we think that there are possible learnings from the field of community-based disaster risk reduction in dealing with communicable diseases. In that, this section unpacks some of the foundational concepts and ideas of community-based disaster risk reduction.

*Table 6.1* Disaster Terminology

| No | Terminology | Definition |
|----|-------------|------------|
| 01 | Capacity | The combination of all the strengths, attributes, and resources available within an organization, community, or society to manage and reduce disaster risks and strengthen resilience. |
| 02 | Disaster | A serious disruption of the functioning of a community or a society at any scale due to hazardous events interacting with conditions of exposure, vulnerability, and capacity, leading to one or more of the following: human, material, economic and environmental losses, and impacts. |
| 03 | Disaster risks | The potential loss of life, injury, or destroyed or damaged assets which could occur to a system, society, or a community in a specific period of time, determined probabilistically as a function of hazard, exposure, vulnerability, and capacity. |
| 04 | Hazard | A process, phenomenon or human activity that may cause loss of life, injury or other health impacts, property damage, social and economic disruption, or environmental degradation. Hazards may be natural, anthropogenic, or socio-natural in origin. |
| 05 | Exposure | The situation of people, infrastructure, housing, production capacities and other tangible human assets located in hazard-prone areas. |
| 06 | Mitigation | The lessening or minimizing of the adverse impacts of a hazardous event. |
| 07 | Preparedness | The knowledge and capacities developed by governments, response and recovery organizations, communities, and individuals to effectively anticipate, respond to, and recover from the impacts of likely, imminent, or current disasters. |
| 08 | Resilience | The ability of a system, community, or society exposed to hazards to resist, absorb, accommodate, adapt to, transform, and recover from the effects of a hazard in a timely and efficient manner, including through the preservation and restoration of its essential basic structures and functions through risk management. |
| 09 | Risk management | Policies and strategies to prevent new risks, reduce existing risks, and manage residual risk, contributing to the strengthening of resilience and reduction of disaster losses. |
| 10 | Vulnerability | The conditions determined by physical, social, economic, and environmental factors or processes which increase the susceptibility of an individual, a community, assets, or systems to the impacts of hazards. |

*Source:* UNDRR (2023).

The approaches of community-based disaster risk reduction acknowledge that in any disaster situation, where pre, during, and post, the communities themselves are the first responders. According to the Capacity for Disaster Reduction Initiative (CaDRi 2020), community-based disaster risk reduction or risk management is a process that communities that are vulnerable to hazards are actively engaged in the identification, analysis, planning, implementation, and evaluation of risk reduction activities. This means that communities are at the centre of decision-making of disaster risk reduction activities, take ownership and responsibility, and are accountable at all stages.

It is important to point out that community-based disaster risk reduction does not take the responsibility and duties of governments away. However, the government authorities and other responsible stakeholders must acknowledge and allow the community ownership of their own lives and their capabilities in dealing with disaster risks. According to O'Keefe et al. (2015) the top-down approaches to dealing with disasters have failed to address the specific local community needs within vulnerabilities, ignore the potential local capabilities, resources, and skills, as well as in many cases increase vulnerabilities. In that, community-based disaster risk reduction can facilitate communities to use their capabilities and resources to better prepare for disasters and adopt mechanisms to reduce their vulnerabilities.

The following are two examples of community-based disaster risk reduction from Cuba (ReliefWeb 2015), and Vietnam (CaDRi 2020).

### *Risk reduction management centres in Cuba*

In response to hydro-meteorological threats, the Cuban government has collaborated with UNDP Cuba and UNDP's Caribbean Risk Management Initiative since 2005 to create the Risk Reduction Management Centre (RRMC), a model of local risk reduction management. At the heart of the model is the promotion of local-level decision-making that relies on coordinated early warning systems, risk and vulnerability studies, communications systems, effective database management and mapping, geographical information system (GIS), and community preparedness. The Cuban Risk Reduction Management Centre model serves as an instrument to ensure that disaster management and development practices in any given territory are informed by an analysis of risk and vulnerability. In addition, each RRMC supports isolated and far-flung communities that may not have access to information so that they can prepare for an approaching threat. Communities are provided with equipment and training to identify, reduce, and communicate risk, as well as take effective protective measures. Between 2005 and 2015, Cuba has been affected by 15 tropical cyclones, of which 11 were classified as hurricanes. In this period, Cuba's Civil Defence system, supported by the RRMC at a local level, has protected more than eight million people, evacuated more than 47,000 tourists, and relocated three settlements.

*Mangrove plantation initiative in Vietnam*

This is an initiative of the Vietnam Red Cross Society, Ministry of Agriculture and Rural Development, and the Ministry of National Resources and Environment across eight coastal provinces in northern Viet Nam. In addition to the protection benefits of mangroves plantation against typhoons and flood risk, as well as climate change impact (reduced disaster-induced losses to public infrastructure, buildings, crops, livestock, aquaculture, reduced costs in sea-dyke maintenance), this CBDRM initiative brought multiple co-benefits to coastal communities (increase aqua culture product revenues, honeybee farming, mangroves carbon value). The two main success criteria are the special attention dedicated to building local capacity and ownership of plantation and maintenance of mangrove forests, and equally important the strong support and commitment on the part of the local government to sustain these efforts.

## Communicable diseases and community-based approaches: Sri Lanka and Cuba

Both Sri Lanka and Cuba are island countries. Both countries have been struggling with various social, political, economic, cultural, and environmental challenges. One of the historical and contemporary similarities between Sri Lanka and Cuba is that both the countries have invested much on public health, and especially introduced community-based approaches to disease control. This section does not attempt to evaluate these approaches, however, attempting to tease out lessons from both Sri Lanka and Cuba in understanding community-based approaches to dealing with communicable diseases.

Both epidemiologically, and demographically, Sri Lanka is in a transition stage. The rapidly aging population and non-communicable diseases have become major causes of mortality and morbidity. Although, suffered through major infectious disease burden, including malaria and TB, Sri Lanka managed to overcome the burden of communicable diseases due to strategic investments in public health and community health. Risk reduction chapter - According to Sri Lanka's National Strategic Plan for the Prevention of Malaria Re-introduction (2018-2022), the country's immunization coverage exceeds 98%.

According to the Government of Sri Lanka (2018), the vision of the Ministry of Health is a healthier nation that contributes to its economic, social, mental, and spiritual development. This vision is supported by a mission to contribute to social and economic development of Sri Lanka by achieving the highest attainable health status through promotive, preventive, curative, and rehabilitative services of high quality made available and accessible to the people of Sri Lanka. The objectives of the Sri Lankan Ministry of Health are as follows:

- To empower the community for maintaining and promoting their health
- To improve comprehensive health services delivery actions

- To strengthen stewardship management functions
- To improve the management of human resources in the health sector

There are very specific objectives for the involvement of communities in dealing with health and well-being. Through the leadership of the Ministry of Health, the regional health services and other health-related sectors including communities are supporting various health programmes by conducting advocacy, behaviour change communication, and social mobilization for health action. In that, the Ministry of Health leads the assistance and development of information, education, and communication (IEC) and behaviour change communication (BCC) materials for health promotion. Further, there are educational and public health interventions on public health issues, to enable to increase control over and promote individual and community health. Finally, the Ministry of Health is conducting and supporting research related to community health and social mobilization.

Figure 6.1 shows the organizational structure of Ministry of Health in Sri Lanka.

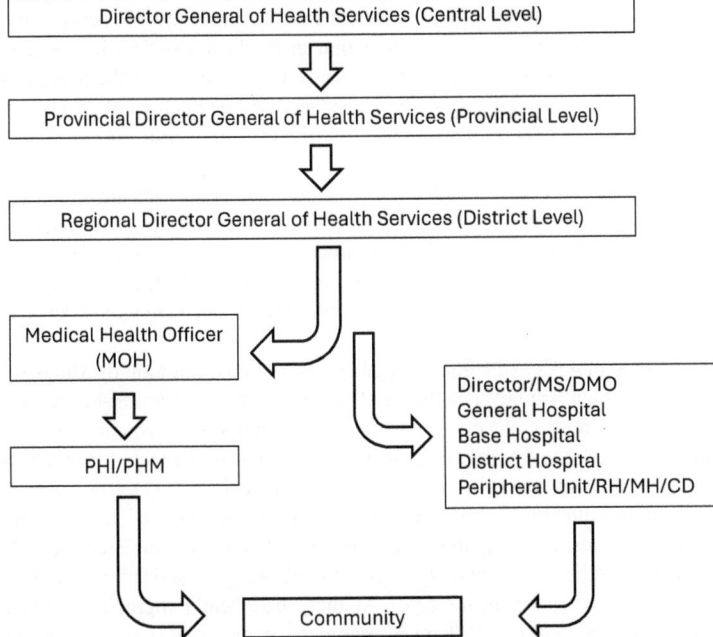

*Figure 6.1* Organizational structure of Ministry of Health, Sri Lanka

Although, a top-down approach, the Public Health Inspectors and Public Health Midwives play a significant role in promoting health within communities. There are many community-based educational campaigns conducted through Public Health Inspectors and Public Health Midwives in collaboration with schools, community organizations, and other stakeholders.

Similar to Sri Lanka, Cuba has many challenges in development. However, the public health in Cuba has many distinctive features. Although economics is an important determinant of population health, Cuba does not correspond to this relationship. In 1959, the Cuban revolution inherited a health system, with a single university hospital and medical school alongside a basic public sector and strong and dominant private health sector (Feinsilver 1993; Ministry of Public Health 1996). Much of the early emphasis was placed on improving basic public health, including sanitation, immunization, and extending medical care into rural areas (Feinsilver 1993). Towards 1980s, the system oriented towards primary care and educating a large number of family doctors. By the 1990s, a family physician and a nurse lived in every block and provided care for 120–160 families (Ministry of Public Health 1996).

What is important and relevant to this book is that the Government of Cuba considers healthcare is a right, which is available to all equally and free of charge (Ministry of Public Health 1996). In an integrated preventative and curative service, public participation in the health system has become vital (Keck and Reed 2012). What is really important is that the healthcare activities are integrated with social and economic development of the country (Demers et al. 1993). Further, Figure 6.2 provides an overview of the Cuban healthcare model.

According to Figure 6.2, the family doctor and nurse teams are an integral part of their communities, where their work is both supported and evaluated by community members. Further, communities become an essential resource for family doctor and nurse teams in organizing and conducting health education events, vaccination camps, mosquito control, and various preventative activities.

Both Sri Lanka and Cuba are signatories to the Declaration of Alma-Ata, which is about primary healthcare. This Declaration is significant, because there is a strong connection between health and socioeconomic development. Second, the fourth article of the Declaration stated that, "people have the right and duty to participate individually and collectively in the planning and implementation of their health care", and the seventh article stated that primary health care "requires and promotes maximum community and individual self-reliance and participation in the planning, organization, operation and control of primary health care". All these are essential ingredients of policymaking and delivery of them in promoting community-based approaches to health and well-being. Further, the guiding principles of the Sendai Framework for Disaster Risk Reduction (2015) point out that, disaster risk reduction

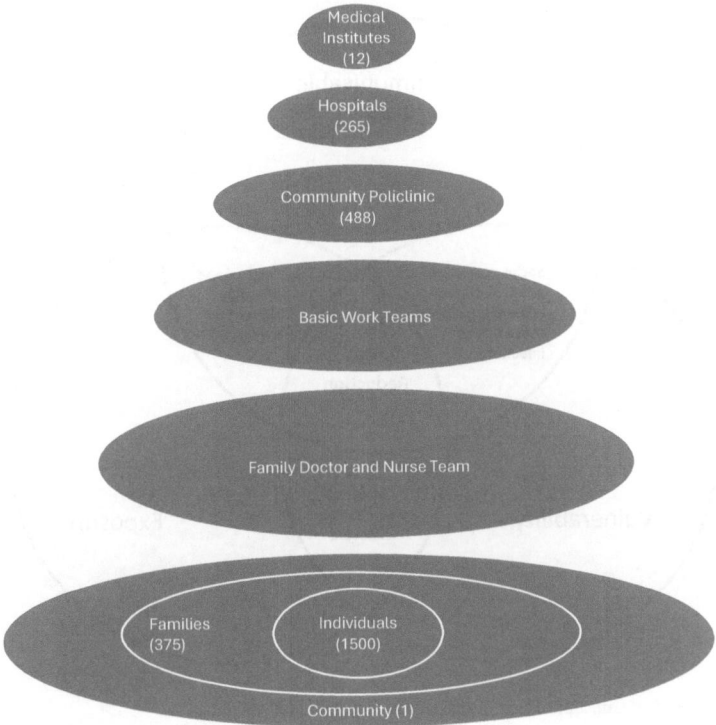

*Figure 6.2* The Cuban health pyramid

requires an all-of-society engagement and partnership. This is where health and risk reduction meet, and through the examples of Sri Lanka and Cuba, it is possible to bring risk reduction into community-based promotion of health and well-being.

Figure 6.3 shows what we have borrowed from disaster risk reduction based on community-based health and well-being approaches from Sri Lanka and Cuba. This diagram was originally presented in the IPCC (2012).

As presented in previous chapters, especially the realities from Papua New Guinea, India, and Bangladesh, communicable diseases such as TB are strongly linked to social, economic, political, cultural, and environmental context where people live. If someone is living in an urban slum in Bangladesh, their sensitivity to infections is higher than someone living in a housing complex with modern facilities. The higher the sensitivity to infection, the higher the vulnerability. Women migrant in Papua New Guinea might not be able to go to daily work due to their vulnerability, which in return decrease their quality of life. This affects their exposure to the infection. This is where

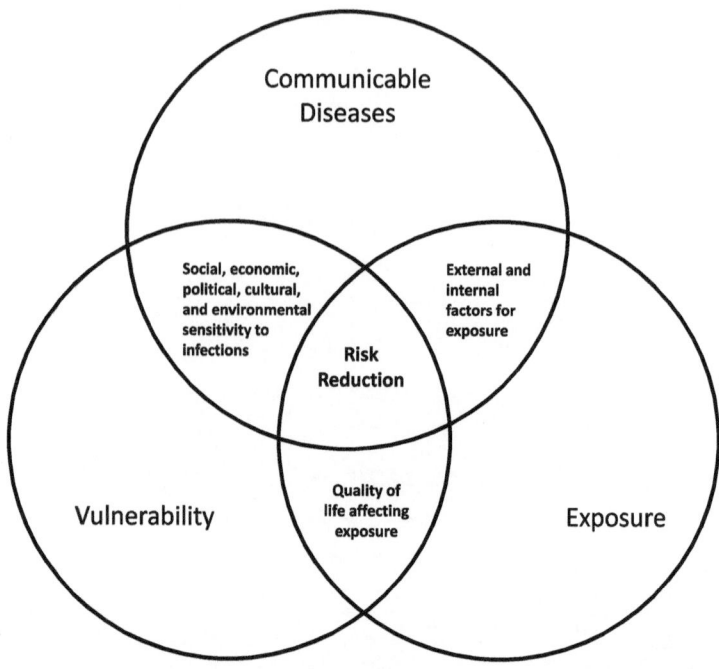

*Figure 6.3* Concept of risk reduction for communicable diseases

the external and internal factors play a role. External factors could be the level of water and sanitation hygiene or air quality. Internal factors could be understood as genetics, co-morbidities, and access to healthy diet. Altogether, Figure 6.3 shows the point where risk reduction must be understood in communicable diseases.

## Proposed framework for communicable disease risk reduction

Based on the above explanation and analysis, we offer a framework for communicable disease risk reduction. This is by no means a rejection of valuable medical interventions or existing healthcare interventions on communicable diseases. However, this proposal is to strengthen the existing efforts and follow the directions of the Declaration of Alma-Ata, especially the 4th and 7th Articles.

This proposed framework is also about horizontal learning from different disciplines. In this case, the health and well-being systems in countries could learn from the field of disaster risk reduction. Like diseases and illnesses, the human populations have been dealing with various hazards and

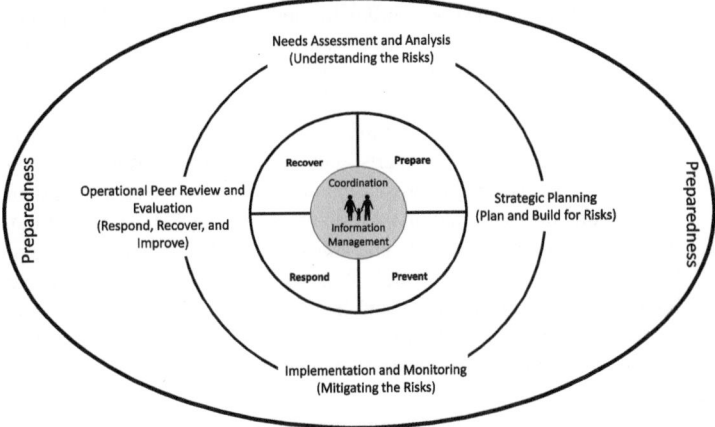

*Figure 6.4* Communicable disease risk reduction framework

disasters. Both the disciplines can learn from each other, and in this instance, the empowerment of communities and bringing them into planning, delivering, managing, monitoring, and evaluating communicable disease risk reduction processes as equal partners of change will increase the effectiveness and impact. Figure 6.4 presents the adaptation of humanitarian programme cycle into dealing with the risks of communicable diseases.

The actions in the framework are described below, and they are all inter-connected. This must be understood and managed in a unified manner using a logical approach within the context. What works in Papua New Guinea may not work in India or Bangladesh. The social, political, cultural, economic, and environmental context must be analysed in collaboration with the community in adapting this framework. The community must be the centre of coordination and information management in the process of implementing this framework. It is very important to establish transparency and accountability to ensure equal participation of the community.

- Preparedness is a paramount element of, and underpins, the entire framework. There are many different types of preparedness. Bottom-up, the practical preparedness is equally important as the top-down, the policy preparedness.
- In collaboration with communities, timely and coordinated assessments and analysis facilitate to identify the needs and provide evidence for planning effective and impactful risk reduction measures. This is about understanding the risks. Communities who have been living through their context must be treated as experts with academics, researchers, policymakers, and other stakeholders must collaborate with them.

- Strategic planning must be coordinated and collaborative with communities. This will help formulation of strategic objectives, what needs to be done to meet them, and what resources (external and internal) are needed to achieve them.
- Through allocated resources, implementation must be done as a collaboration between technical experts, and communities. In some cases, the technical expertise can be found within communities – such as traditional medical practitioners, traditional birth attendants, and students. Monitoring of agreed outputs and outcome indicators can facilitate the next step.
- Operational peer review of the risk reduction process can be evaluated both by external stakeholders and internal stakeholders. This evaluative element can strengthen the risk reduction and will establish a cycle of assessment, planning, implementation, and evaluation.

While implementation of the risk reduction framework must be flexible and adaptable to different contexts, it must at a minimum address the above elements. This proposed framework must sit within the national health policies, healthcare systems, and various stakeholders such as educational institutes, livelihood authorities, and environmental departments. This framework can be adapted to compliment or build on existing structures. This communicable disease risk reduction framework must contribute to building existing capabilities, capacities, and resilience of communities against different types of diseases.

## Conclusion

The famous Bengali proverb, জলে কুমীর, ডাঙ্গায় বাঘ (which translates to a tiger on the land, a crocodile in the water), means that a person is stuck between two extreme risks. As this book explained, TB or any other communicable disease creates double-bind challenges to most communities in the Global South. Poverty, which creates difficulties to maintain health and well-being can be the tiger on the land. The suffering induced through communicable diseases such as TB can be the crocodile in the water.

What we suggest through our proposed framework is the communities that are suffering from poverty and vulnerable to communicable disease risks must be at the centre of any preparedness, response, prevention, and recovery. This involvement by the community would allow them to become equal partners of change in communicable disease risk reduction processes, as well as engage with overall development processes.

While recognizing the devastating impacts of TB, and many other forms of communicable diseases, we point towards community-owned processes, that must be discussed, designed, delivered, monitored, and evaluated within the context of development. Any efforts to tackle communicable diseases from a single discipline analysis have failed over the past 70 years, and we must bring different approaches, frameworks, and concepts that are useful to people.

# References

Capacity for Disaster Reduction Initiative. (2020) *Compendium of Good Practices on Community Based Disaster Risk Management*. Geneva: UNDP.

Demers, R.V., Kemble, S., Orris, M. and Orris, P. (1993) Family practice in Cuba: evolution into the 1990s. *Family Practice*, 10(2), 164–168.

Feinsilver, J.M. (1993) *Healing the Masses. Cuban Health Politics at Home and Abroad*. Berkely: University of California Press.

Holtz, D., Markham, A., Cell, K. and Ekwurzel, B. (2014) *National Landmarks at Risk: How Rising Seas, Floods, and Wildfires Are Threatening the United States' Most Cherished Historic Sites*. Washington, DC: Union of Concerned Scientists.

Intergovernmental Panel on Climate Change (IPCC). (2012) *Managing the Risks of Extreme Events and Disasters to Advance Climate Change Adaptation. A Special Report of Working Groups I and II of the Intergovernmental Panel on Climate Change*, edited by C.B. Field, V. Barros, T.F. Stocker, D. Qin, D.J. Dokken, K.L. Ebi, M.D. Mastrandrea, K.J. Mach, G.-K. Plattner, S.K. Allen, M. Tignor, and P.M. Midgley. Cambridge, UK and New York, NY: Cambridge University Press.

Jayasekara, R., Siriwardana, C., Amaratunga, D. and Haigh, R. (2021) Analysing the effectiveness of varied stakeholder segments in preparedness planning for epidemics and pandemics in Sri Lanka: application of social network analysis (SNA). In *COVID 19: Impact, Mitigation, Opportunities and Building Resilience: From Adversity to Serendipity*. National Science Foundation of Sri Lanka, pp. 540–553.

Keck, C.W. and Reed, G.A. (2012) The curious case of Cuba. *American Journal of Public Health*, 102(8), e13–e22.

Ministry of Health – Anti Malaria Campaign. (2018) *National Strategic Plan for Prevention of Re-introduction of Malaria in Sri Lanka 2018–2022*. Colombo: Government of Sri Lanka.

Ministry of Public Health. (1996) Analysis of the Health Sector in Cuba (Ministerio de Salud Publica. Analisis del Sector Salud en Cuba. Con la colaboracion OMS/OPS.) Havana, Cuba, Available at: https://salud.msp.gob.cu/documents, accessed on May 07, 2024.

O'Keefe, P., O'Brien, G. and Jayawickrama, J. (2015) Disastrous disasters: a polemic on capitalism, climate change and humanitarianism. In A. Collins, S. Jones, S.B. Manyena, J. Jayawickrama (Eds.), *Natural Hazards, Risks, and Disasters in Society: A Cross-Disciplinary Overview*, Elsevier's Hazards and Disasters Series. Oxford: Elsevier, pp. 34–43.

O'keefe, P., Westgate, K. and Wisner, B. (1976) Taking the naturalness out of natural disasters. *Nature*, 260(5552), 566–567.

ReliefWeb. (2015) A Cuban Model for a Resilient Caribbean. Geneva, UNDP. Available at: https://reliefweb.int/report/cuba/cuban-model-resilient-caribbean, accessed on April 17, 2024.

Smith, N. (2006) There's no such thing as a natural disaster. Understanding Katrina: perspectives from the social sciences, 11, SSRI. Available at: https://projects.iq.harvard.edu/files/retreat/files/smith_2006_theres_no_such_thing.pdf, accessed on May 30, 2024.

United Nations. (2015) Disaster Risk Reduction Terminology. Available at: https://www.undrr.org/drr-glossary/terminology, accessed on: April 12, 2024.

United Nations. (2015) *Sendai Framework for Disaster Risk Reduction: 2015–2030*. Geneva: United Nations Office for Disaster Risk Reduction.

United Nations. (2023) *The Humanitarian Programme Cycle*. Geneva: UN Office for the Coordination of Humanitarian Affairs (UN OCHA).

World Health Organisation. (1978) Declaration of Alma-Ata: International Conference on Primary Health Care, Alma-Ata, USSR, September 6–12, 1978. https://www.who.int/teams/social-determinants-of-health/declaration-of-alma-ata accessed on May 07, 2024.

# 7 Conclusion

*Arnab Chakraborty, Janaka Jayawickrama, and Yong-an Zhang*

This book is interdisciplinary in nature, and while the way of writing conclusions of books or articles differ in diverse social science disciplines, we would try and keep this in sync with the rest of this work. In fact, with tuberculosis (TB), it is easier to do that, since the history of TB is an ongoing process, which we are still experiencing and getting affected by in our daily lives. This book takes a historical approach to compiling contemporary literature, examining how scholars have historically viewed tuberculosis (TB). Additionally, it adopts an ethnographic-anthropological perspective to explore human resilience and the struggle against the disease.

Chapter 3 on Papua New Guinea explains the challenges of an individual journey, within complex decisions, desperate measures, and profound sacrifices one must make in a resource-poor setting when dealing with a communicable disease such as TB. Chapter 4 on India explains the challenges that a national TB programme faced within a complex social, political, and economic context through a historical lens. Chapter 5 on Bangladesh takes us through the local community health workers and how it implements the global health policies in a developing country. Combined with Chapter 2, which provides a historiography of TB, Chapter 6 points towards the importance of investing in risk reduction while other existing interventions continue. All these chapters are a combination of the disciplines of history, anthropology, global health, disaster studies, and human geography.

This book is one of the first to highlight the significance of interdisciplinary approaches in understanding global health research. It offers an alternative to traditional top-down or bottom-up methodologies, encouraging new ways of analyzing, critiquing, and communicating global health issues. This book takes multi-pronged approaches to understand the nature of this disease and how negotiation, collaboration, recognition among community workers can go a long way towards handling any global health crises. Thinking historically encourages us to engage with historical materials in the way a historian would, analyzing sources critically and understanding context to form a deeper comprehension of events and processes.

DOI: 10.4324/9781032634647-7

While coming to the end of completing this book, we realize there is still a lot of work to be done on TB, and we are living this history. Throughout the book, we have underscored the enduring significance of this disease and the diverse strategies employed to combat it. TB even today remains a global health challenge, reflecting a complex interplay of historical, cultural, and socio-economic factors. Our exploration has revealed the critical importance of integrating scientific advancements with community-based interventions and public awareness campaigns. The varying experiences from different regions highlight that while biomedical solutions like the DOTS strategy have made significant strides, they must be complemented by local engagement and tailored, holistic approaches to be truly effective.

As we move forward, it is imperative to continue fostering interdisciplinary research and international collaboration to address the multifaceted nature of TB. Future efforts should focus on not only improving medical treatments and healthcare infrastructure but also understanding the socio-cultural dimensions of the disease. By learning from past successes and failures, and by continuously adapting our strategies to the evolving landscape of global health, we can make meaningful progress in the fight against tuberculosis. This book serves as a call to action for researchers, policymakers, and healthcare professionals to remain vigilant and innovative in their efforts to eradicate this ancient yet persistent disease.

The COVID-19 pandemic has led to the reallocation of healthcare resources in the Global South, where health systems are often under-resourced and overburdened. Medical staff, diagnostic facilities, and financial resources have been diverted to manage the COVID-19 crisis, resulting in reduced capacity for TB diagnosis and treatment. Clinics and hospitals have faced overwhelming patient loads, limiting their ability to provide consistent care for TB patients. Lockdowns and movement restrictions have severely impacted TB patients' ability to access healthcare services. In many areas, public transportation shutdowns and curfews have made it difficult for patients to reach medical facilities for regular check-ups and medication refills. This disruption has led to treatment interruptions, increasing the risk of drug resistance and disease transmission within communities.

Furthermore, the economic fallout from the pandemic has disproportionately affected low-income populations in the Global South, many of whom are at higher risk of TB. Job losses and reduced incomes have made it harder for individuals to afford healthcare services and nutritious food, which is critical for TB patients' recovery. The compounded impact of economic and health crises has deepened the inequities faced by TB patients. The pandemic has also highlighted the importance of community-based health interventions in the Global South. With healthcare facilities stretched thin, community health workers have played a crucial role in maintaining TB care continuity. They have facilitated remote monitoring, medication delivery, and patient education, helping to mitigate some of the pandemic's adverse effects on TB treatment. In fact, COVID-19 has worked as a trigger for a lot of people, and it made people develop active TB from its latent form. With lockdowns, low nutrition, and congested apartments aided by unhygienic places in the developing countries, TB kept ticking as a time-bomb only to manifest its form aided by the recent pandemic outbreak.

Innovative approaches have emerged as a response to these challenges. The use of digital health technologies, such as telemedicine, mobile health platforms, and digital adherence monitoring, has been pivotal in ensuring that TB patients continue to receive care. These technologies have allowed for remote consultations and support, reducing the need for in-person visits and minimizing the risk of COVID-19 exposure. In conclusion, the COVID-19 pandemic has underscored the fragility and resilience of TB control efforts in the Global South. While the pandemic has disrupted healthcare systems and exacerbated challenges, it has also spurred innovation and highlighted the critical role of community-based interventions. By integrating these lessons into future TB programmes, we can build more robust and adaptable health systems that are better equipped to handle both ongoing and future health crises. This book emphasizes the interconnectedness of global health challenges and calls for a unified, inclusive approach to combatting TB, particularly in the most vulnerable regions of the world.

The historiography of TB shows that efforts to control the disease have been as much about addressing social and economic inequalities as about medical interventions hence in this book we have taken a multi-pronged approach to elucidate that. During the colonial era, TB spread rapidly due to poor living conditions, malnutrition, and lack of access to medical care among colonized populations. These conditions have persisted in many parts of the world, exacerbated by post-colonial economic policies and globalization, which have often prioritized profit over people's health. Today, TB remains a significant challenge in low- and middle-income countries, where health systems are often under-resourced and overburdened. The disease's persistence is a stark reminder of the need for comprehensive health policies that address the root causes of health inequities. The United Nations Sustainable Development Goals (SDGs), particularly the target of ending the TB epidemic by 2030, provide a crucial framework for addressing these challenges. However, achieving these global targets requires more than biomedical interventions; it necessitates a holistic approach that fosters a harmonious relationship between humans and their environment. The fight against TB is emblematic of broader struggles for social justice and equitable development. Addressing TB effectively demands sustained international cooperation and commitment to tackling the social determinants of health. This includes improving living conditions, ensuring access to nutritious food, and providing comprehensive healthcare that is responsive to the needs of the most vulnerable populations. Moreover, it involves addressing broader issues such as economic inequality, lack of education, and inadequate infrastructure, which contribute to the conditions in which TB thrives.

The relationship between TB and social determinants of health is well-documented. For instance, malnutrition weakens the immune system, making individuals more susceptible to TB infection and disease progression. Similarly, conditions such as diabetes and HIV/AIDS, which are more prevalent in poorer communities, further increase the risk of TB. Unplanned urbanization leads to overcrowded living conditions, which facilitate the spread of TB. Addressing these underlying factors is essential for controlling the disease. The integration of social, political, economic, cultural, and environmental perspectives provides a richer understanding of the contemporary challenges posed by TB. The SDGs offer a framework within which these challenges can be addressed, particularly the target of ending the TB epidemic. However, this chapter argues that achieving these global targets requires more than biomedical interventions; it necessitates a holistic approach that fosters a harmonious relationship between humans and their environment. Environmental factors also play a significant role in the persistence of TB. For example, indoor air pollution, often a result of cooking with solid fuels in poorly ventilated homes, increases the risk of TB. Improving housing conditions and reducing exposure to indoor pollutants can help mitigate this risk. Similarly, ensuring access to clean water and sanitation can prevent the spread of infections that can weaken the immune system and make individuals more susceptible to TB.

Moreover, the economic impact of TB is profound. The disease predominantly affects individuals in their most productive years, leading to significant economic losses for families and communities. Lost income, medical expenses, and the long-term health effects of TB can drive families further into poverty, creating a vicious cycle of disease and poverty. Breaking this cycle requires not only medical treatment but also economic support for affected individuals and communities. The fight against TB also demands attention to cultural factors. Stigma and discrimination against TB patients can prevent individuals from seeking timely diagnosis and treatment. Educational campaigns to raise awareness about TB, its transmission, and its treatment are crucial for reducing stigma and encouraging people to seek care. Community engagement and culturally sensitive approaches are essential for ensuring that TB control efforts are effective and sustainable. The global health community has made significant strides in TB research and treatment over the past decades. Advances in diagnostic techniques, such as molecular testing, have improved the accuracy and speed of TB diagnosis. New treatments and drug regimens have been developed to combat drug-resistant TB, a growing concern in many parts of the world. However, these medical advances must be accompanied by efforts to strengthen health systems and ensure that all individuals have access to quality care.

International cooperation is essential for addressing the global TB epidemic. This includes funding for TB programmes, research collaborations, and sharing of best practices. The Global Fund to Fight AIDS, Tuberculosis and Malaria, for example, has been instrumental in supporting TB control efforts in low- and middle-income countries. The holistic approach would only work if we start involving more people on the ground, the national offices, local funders, and people who are willing to help. We need a collaborative effort, and the WHO or any global health organizations would need to connect with those locally involved in making a difference. Those without getting funding from global organizations or credit in Western-centric reports and literature need to be celebrated and acknowledged for broader cooperation, including South-South cooperation. Achieving the global targets for TB control also requires addressing broader issues of global health governance. This includes ensuring that health policies are inclusive and equitable, and that they prioritize the needs of the most vulnerable populations. It also involves advocating for policies that address the social determinants of health and promote sustainable development. Ultimately, the fight against TB is a fight for social justice. It is about ensuring that all individuals, regardless of their socio-economic status or geographic location, have the opportunity to live healthy and productive lives. This holistic development paradigm not only targets the disease but also promotes overall human well-being, aligning closely with the aspirations of the SDGs for a healthier, more equitable world.

TB's prevalence in regions facing political instability, migration crises, and environmental challenges, such as climate change, exemplifies how health issues are intertwined with socio-political and environmental factors. The displacement of populations due to conflict or climate-induced disasters often leads to overcrowded living conditions and strained healthcare services, creating fertile ground for TB transmission. In tackling TB, we must adopt a holistic approach that addresses these interconnected global problems. Strengthening health systems, ensuring equitable access to care, and fostering international cooperation are essential steps. By learning from the history of TB and understanding its current context, we can develop comprehensive strategies that not only aim to eradicate TB but also enhance our overall resilience against global health threats. This book serves as a call to action to view TB not in isolation, but as part of the broader tapestry of challenges that define our contemporary world, urging a united and multifaceted response.

This book is located within Asia and the Pacific region. However, what we discuss in this book does not limit to the region. Most countries in Africa, Latin/South America, and West Asia (or the Middle East from a Western point of understanding) are suffering from various forms of communicable diseases that are strongly connected to poverty and underdevelopment. We understand the importance of the debates and discussions that must arise from these countries where people become equal partners of change in reducing the risks of communicable diseases as well as their overall development.

# Index